CANNABIS USE SURVEY

CANNABIS USE SURVEY

Confessions, Insights, and Opinions

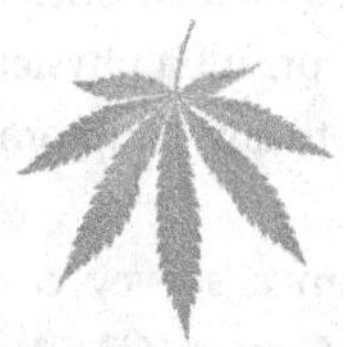

LAURIE K MISCHLEY ND PHD MPH

Bastyr University

MICHELLE SEXTON ND

The Cannabis and Social Policy Center (CASP)

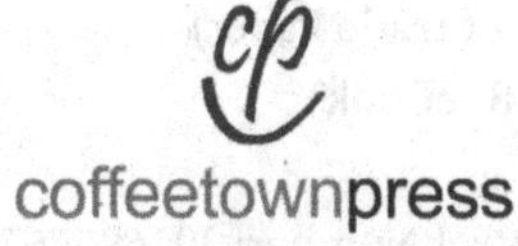

Seattle, WA

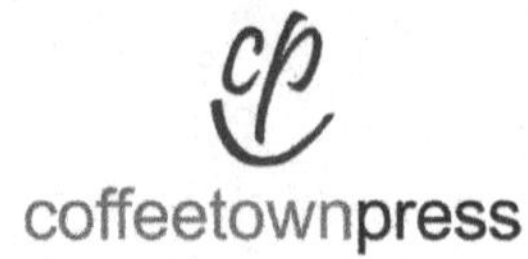

Coffeetown Press
PO Box 70515
Seattle, WA 98127

For more information go to: www.coffeetownpress.com
www.CannabisSurvey.org

The following is not intended as a substitute for the medical advice of physicians. The reader should regularly consult a physician in matters relating to his/her health and particularly with respect to any symptoms that may require diagnosis or medical attention.
These are actual results from a survey conducted by Bastyr University and the Cannabis and Social Policy Center (CASP), designed and implemented by Laurie K. Mischley and Michelle Sexton. Spelling and grammar errors have been left uncorrected to retain the flavor of the original responses. All identifying information has been redacted.

Cover design by Sabrina Sun
Cover photograph by Michelle Sexton
Photo of Michelle Sexton by Sam Sabzehzar

ISBN: 978-1-60381-615-1 (Trade Paper)
ISBN: 978-1-60381-616-8 (eBook)

Library of Congress Control Number: 2016957678
Printed in the United States of America

Welcome to the "Cannabis Use Survey."

You are eligible to participate if you have used Cannabis at least once in the past 90 days.

Your participation in this survey is completely anonymous. No information you provide can or will tell us who you are. You may skip any questions you do not want to answer. By continuing to complete this survey, you agree to have the information that you provide used for research purposes by the identified investigators at Bastyr University. It will take approximately 10-20 minutes to complete the survey.

The information you provide will help inform physicians, researchers, policy-makers, and patients about the potential risks and/or benefits of Cannabis as a therapeutic or recreational agent.

Please direct any questions or concerns you may have about this survey to lmischley@bastyr.edu.

Please direct any questions you have about your rights as a research subject to David Hammond, PhD at the Bastyr University Office of Research Integrity: irb@bastyr.edu.

We appreciate your time and honesty.

Investigators:

Laurie Mischley, ND, PhD, MPH
lmischley@bastyr.edu

Michelle Sexton, ND
msextonnd@cannabisandsocialpolicy.org

Introduction

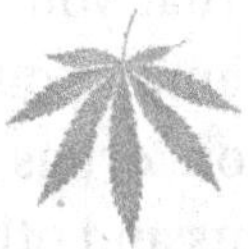

Do you struggle with the concept of an "evil weed" having the potential to heal? Do you have friends or family who use cannabis and you don't understand why? Are you wondering if cannabis might be for you? Or, maybe you are asking yourself if your love of cannabis is addiction?

If any of these questions resonate with you, then this book is for you. In these pages you will read firsthand accounts of people who have a relationship with cannabis/marijuana/pot. While this may seem ridiculous to some, for those in this relationship, it is no joke. People who used cannabis as a "recreation" in the past now turn to it as a pain reliever. Those who struggle with anxiety or depression find an altered consciousness that invokes creativity and peace. Some describe their struggle with the "stigma" associated with cannabis use. Some are in a covert relationship because it is not legal where they live.

The Cannabis Use Survey is the largest of its kind, in peer-reviewed publication, and was born from our curiosity about this mushrooming phenomenon of cannabis/human relationships. At the end of the questions that comprise our data, we invited our survey participants to tell us "anything that you think we should know". You may find yourself somewhere within these pages.

Beyond this voice, these stories point to a larger narrative, that of dissatisfaction with how healthcare is being delivered and the fallacy of single molecule medicine. It is estimated that 80% of the world's population still use herbs as a part of "traditional medicine." The National Center for Complimentary and Integrative Health reports that Americans spend $30 billion a year, out-of-pocket on several "complimentary" approaches to health. Pain is one of the leading reasons that Americans turn to both cannabis and alternative approaches.

The default medical-establishment position continues to be that if it's not a synthetic pill manufactured in a pill factory, it can't be medicine. Most of the stories that you read here beg to differ. Plants are the original medicine and among our responders, 60% report that they have replaced prescription drugs with cannabis: opiates, anti-inflammatories, anti-depressants and others. If you are struggling with a poor quality of life related to prescription drugs these stories are for you.

People love pot. Is this safe? Does it work? Is this legal? Answers may vary. We invite you, the reader to decide for yourself.

—Dr. Michelle Sexton

I GREW UP IN A SMALL NORTHERN Michigan town where I was taught, by teachers and parents I trusted, not to use drugs. I was taught that cannabis was a gateway drug, and it was just a matter of time before cannabis use would lead to cocaine and heroin. I was taught that only losers use drugs. Good kids, those who would make something of their life, remained drug-free.

By high school, I began witnessing alcohol leading to belligerence, senseless fights, and regrettable sexual encounters. I watched cocaine and heroin consume friends' lives. Weed … well, I saw cannabis users playing sports, making art, participating in Youth in Government, Latin club, student counsel, and making honor role.

The incongruence between what I was being taught by trusted authority figures and what I was observing for myself got under my skin. By college, I was determined to do my part to remedy the miscommunication between those who used cannabis and those who judged it. So here I am, fulfilling an academic dream that began in 1989. Cannabis research is not my career—it is my curiosity.

We realize that the way this book is organized will be confusing to some readers. No subject headings, just numbered responses. By providing the responses this way, we hoped to convey the *tremendous* diversity of the human experience. The messy complexity is part of what we want to communicate.

People within our community have responded positively to the numbering, which allows them to highlight their favorite. "Did you see what # 227 said?" We're looking forward to hearing readers' responses and using them to further the conversation. Perhaps we'll even start a book club or do a sequel.

This is a biased survey. Those who have tried cannabis and had a negative experience and those who have failed to derive pleasure from the plant are not represented here. This is a study of individuals who chose to use the plant. We are simply asking "Why?"

In this book we draw no conclusions, we simply give voice to those who have been underground. These are the sentiments of your friends, family, and co-workers who use and are afraid to discuss it with you for fear of judgment and retribution. Here, we play messenger.

Fellow researchers, please contact us if you'd like to expand this survey or access existing data.

Cannabis users, this survey is ongoing. Please consider visiting the study website (www.CannabisSurvey.org) and participating. The more people that participate, the more we learn.

—Dr. Laurie K. Michley

OUR GOAL IS TO BETTER UNDERSTAND THE MEDICAL AND RECREATIONAL USE OF MARIJUANA. PLEASE TELL US ANYTHING YOU THINK WE SHOULD KNOW.

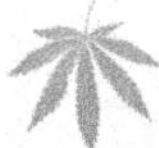

1. I first tried marijuana when I was 21 years old. Now, 46 years later, I still smoke pot. I am 67 years old and have not taken a prescription medication in over 30 years. Has regular cannabis use enabled this? I have no idea. I am active...hiking, canoeing, camping, bicycling. My last hike was 11.5 miles... to the Confluence Overlook in Canyonlands Natl Park. Has cannabis enabled this? I don't know. I do know that I am living proof that prohibitionist propaganda is a fallacy...a blatant lie. The worst experience I ever had with cannabis was spending 5 years in Federal Prison for a marijuana offense.

2. Home grown cannabis is safer because I can control how strong the THC content is. Buying from an unknown source can sometimes lead to cannabis that has been compromised with substances to increase weight. I am not able to grow at home because of the legal status of the drug in this country. Stupid idiotic and ignorant politicians stand in the way of progress again. Thank you.

3. i am a medical user who finds effective relief from chronic pain

and associated depression and anxiety. lack of affordable legal access and federal laws prohibiting what my state law would permit me, as a qualifying patient, to do, that is, grow my own medicine at home, make it impossible for me to access cannabis in anything but illegal ways. the stigma of criminality contributes to my sense of being marginalized and at risk of losing freedom and life support systems simply for using the safest remedial approach to managing my conditions i have ever been able to find.

4. I have relied exclusively on raw cannabis to relieve my symptoms since 1994. It doesn't work for everybody but it works for me.

5. I use cannabis because it's fun. It allows me think in an unusual way for a few hours before returning to reality. It also increases my ability to appreciate movies, books, music etc. In addition, it can sometimes be a good excuse to get together with a group of friends and just hang out and have fun.

6. Interesting survey! I foundmy read on some questions is very ambiguous. it is a start. Like the timing on the short term????intervals and method of absorption,etc.

7. It really depends on what kind of person you are. I was raised around cannabis, so I almost find it in the norm for me. It's truly not a big deal for me, but for others, it seems to be harder for them to cope with the effects of it.

8. - gives insight into difficult problems - alleviates pain - makes the mundane interesting - potential prevention of Alzheimer's

9. -MARIJUANA IS SOOO GOOD -IT IS NOT ADDICTIVE

-IT SHOULD BE LEGALIZED TO BE GROWN PROPERLY 'ARTIFICIAL' GROW OF CANNABIS IS ADDICTIVE-

10. ;)

11. 'Addiction' to cannabis is mostly mental, but also a bit physiological or psychosomatic. Mostly I just want to smoke it, I almost never (anymore) feel the 'need' for it.

12. 'Have you ever used Cannabis as a substitute for illegal drugs?' I think this is an ambiguous question. If you say no, you could mean that you do not do illicit drugs or that you do and don't use Cannabis as a substitute.

13. 'i dont know' if marijuana is addictive because although never having urges, the sensation of being high or wanting to feel that way does cross your mind. As well, as for if it affects my sleep pattern....I know when im stoned I sleep easy and through the night while when sober I may (not always) struggle to sleep. I do recognize however REM sleep is of higher quality thus sleeping when stoned cannot be as I do not dream. (compared to vivid dreams when sober)

14. 'SHORT TERM EFFECTS' Anxiety and hyperstimulation that I feel when Im on cannabis, that I'm taking to treat anxiety, subside when the high does. Afterwards I am very relaxed, thinking much clearer and more productive. Because of these effects of cannabis, I dont usually smoke it in a social setting and usually smoke it before falling asleep. 'In selecting my Cannabis medicine I consider these to be important factors' Real answer - None if the above. I take what I can manage to get a hold of. It is illegal in my state and they've arrested/stopped all the safe/

high quality growers/dealers. 'Gender' My GENDER is male. I'm female bodied, Im a transman. 'Current Employment' I work over 40 hours a week. I am employed part time- my boss knows I smoke and we both support legalizing cannabis. She cannot afford to give me more hours due to economy. The rest of the hours I am self employed, freelance work. Surveys are too black and white!

15. 1. Recreational retail stores will not have the medicine I need. It has taken me 12 years to create the right strain that works for me. If I can't grow this strain where will I get it? 2. Medical Marijuana dispensaries sell medicine, doesn't make sense to have a Liquor Dept. run medicine, they know nothing about medical access, they used to sell Tequila, and Whiskey not sure how that qualifies someone to make medical decisions and policy. 3. If you force people to buy overpriced medicine that is ineffective, the Drug Cartels will jump in and sell it cheap to anyone who wants it including children. 3. We almost beat the Drug Cartels, but they obviously have influence even at the state level, as this is their Christmas present. The street price of 3.5 grams is $40.00, the Cartels and the dealers have been trying to raise the price and profits for decades, unsuccessfully, however the WA State government is planning to do it for them, Merry Christmas.

16. 1. Due to variations w/in the phenotypes, the short term effects are usually substantially different from strain to strain. 2. The term 'addictive' is subjective. I find that cannnabis improves my overall quality of life, similar to exercise and healthful dietary intake: = lifestyle choice. 3. The wording of whether or not one has been ticketed or in a crash while under the influence of cannabis sounds like an automatic admission of guilt or fault

and does not address the relevance within the situation. 4. I strongly disagree with arbitrary and prohibitively low per se nanogram percentages as an indicator of inebriation or the ability to operate a motor vehicle. Cannabis effects and coordination are not as intrinsically correlated as they are with alcohol.

17. 1) Short-term effects vary enormously for me depending on the strain/variety of cannabis I've used. 2) Cannabis use has a huge and direct correlation for me with decreased use of NSAIDs - my rheumatologist instructed me to take 12 Advil per day for the rest of my life (!!!), but I have consistently had far better results over the past three years smoking 30-40mg cannabis/day and occasionally also having one Tylenol if needed. I can't begin to tell you how grateful I am to my naturopath for authorizing medical cannabis use for me!

18. 11 months ago I had a double mastectomy. I didn't take 1 prescription pain pill or antibiotic after 2 surgeries. Last one in Nov. 2015. I researched and used cannabis, (thc, cbd-isolate.) Used all ways! I also ate very good. All vegan! Juices. Plus, colloidal silver, oregano oil.... Love to tell you more! I journaled. Btw.. Outpatient, I was up the next day making breakfast.

19. 420 blaze it

20. A 30 yr RN, I have researched cannabis and agree, that it is a basic human nutrient. Imbalances in the endocannabinoid system are most likely responsible for the need to 'medicate' or 'recreate.' If we had it in our daily diets, we wouldn't be nearly as sick and our society would be much healthier.

21. A friend described the profound pain relief he experienced after only 2 weeks taking cannabis pills. I did research to help reduce the polyneuropathy I have had for more than 30 years. My symptoms include, constant pain, heat and numbness in my legs, feet, toes, as well as muscle spasm in my back, arms, legs, trigger finger, and periodic electrical-type pains in my legs and toes. The pains make sleep restless and shallow. Without enough sleep, weight regulation and healing are prevented. Using a high CBD and low THC cannabis -- infused in glycerin -- I was able to stop taking ibuprofen, and now rarely take acetaminophen -- both of which have negative effects when taken regularly over long periods of time. I take one large dropper of the CBD infusion in a glass of water before sleep. And a re-dose 3-4 hours later, about half way through sleep. Sometimes will take another dropper full during the day if the pain is searing. Thanks for doing the survey.

22. a lot of how cannabis does is in the head the body shows any sine of withdraws

23. A lot of people tend to rely upon consumable and non-consumable items to get through their days instead of facing deeply rooted issues. Cannabis is just one of these things.

24. A lot of the effects of cannabis depend on the strain you're smoking. At times I am incredibly motivated, and others I can barely be assed to get off the couch. Good luck with your survey!

25. A study on sources of cannabis, ie grower, dispensary, self grow, street dealer might be the only thing that I would think to include.

26. a truly victimless drug.. that benefits its users in multiple ways..

27. A very long time user, going on almost 2 decades. The only negativity surrounding cannabis usage are the legal ramifications brought on by the idiots we have in charge. Cannabis increases the quality of your life and if it were legal, completely legal; to grow, smoke, carry and possess, than the ONLY downside to it will be alleviated, thus making it a perfect enhancement to your life.

28. A very safe pleasureable social and relaxing way of comunicating with self and other like minded people

29. Absolute wonder drug

30. Add in the categories of outdoor vs indoor, and organic vs non-organic

31. Adverse side effects that commonly described throughout media are not side effects of the drug rather the side effects of prohibtion, use of cannabis as a depression alleviation tool (lifting mood when stuck in a depressive state) i have found to be extremely benefical, rather than a continued use of pharmaceutical chemicals which can develop into addictive regions and affecting the ability for different emotions to be expeirinced by the users. cannabis offers a system of help which i feel are benefical not only in terms of mood but in general health.

32. After multiple years of trying other options for my issues, cannabis is the one thing that has helped multiple problems and improved my life.

33. after several failed back surgeries, i became addicted to pain pills, they had me on fentenil, liquid methadone (1800ml). percocette, vicodin and klonazapam. i am lucky to have survived this period in my life. in 2008, i found marijuana again, and tho still a painful life, it is bearable, with pot. i stopped the pain pills, and now i grow my own, make my own topical pain analgesic, and my own concentrates. with medical marijuana, i am able to live a fairly high quality of life.

34. After suddenly losing my father last year, I relied heavily on using weed to help myself not think about the sad feelings I was experiencing all day every day. It helps me function normally without having to effect much else.

35. After using cannabis for medical reasons, I gradually transitioned to a partial medi/rec user after about 4 months of use. I did notice that my symptoms that I were using cannabis to treat (migraines/ nausea) became much worse in a time period of 3 days where I stopped cold-turkey due to location reasons.

36. After using Cannabis for some time my desire for alcohol is now very low and I find myself hardly ever having a drink - when I do it's just one.

37. Alcohol and other drugs (such as Cocaine and Ecstacy) have caused me nothing but problems and depression in the past. I struggle with my mood and my appetite. I don't sleep too well either. Cannabis solves all of that more. It reduces my stress, lets me eat (a lot), makes me enjoy exercise and being outside. There is no reason cannabis should be illegal in any country.

38. All cannabis consumed for medical purposes should be

grown organically without pesticides or synthetic chemicals (hydroponic). Unfortunately this is all that is available on the street, and I believe this is harmful as people are smoking chemicals instead of plant material.

39. ALL Cannabis is good for me, I Smoke it for my depression, its quick relief helps me get through the day. I smoke or Vape it. I use Cannabis Extract oil made with FOOD GRADE Grain Alcohol lke everclear NOT ISO or Naptha (Also known as RSO) I never use RSO. And I use a Salve to run into my joints. My point is MANY of us use it ALL day long everyday and every form of it . I also use THC AND CBDs Because the WHOLE plant has its uses. Not Just smoking. Many patients feel the same only these surveys tend to steer us in the direction you all want to steer us in. Not the way we really use this. NOT ALL PATIENTS Want only CBDs

40. All people allover the world should know about the benefits and positive character of this amazing plant that makes the world into a better place and socializes people from all races

41. All powerful tools contain both the ability to transform/grow and also the potential for abuse/misuse/hinderance.

42. All rhetoric aside, it has changed my life.

43. all that has been done up to now ARE the BIGGEST LIES EVER TOLD--Cannabis is the anti-dote to radiation which is now in major abundance due to Fukishima--time for gov and docs to say sorry for being the assholes THEY have been and get the ACCESS OUT THERE EVERYWHERE NOW!

44. Allot of People Claim Marijuana is Addictive but they can go without. There is No Physical Dependence or Physical Addiction. Marijuana is Not a Hallucinogen, Anyone who Claims to have Seen something Out of this world While under the influence of Cannabis is either Lieing OR the person they purchased their Marijuana from had laced it. If Marijuana were to be legalized & people were allowed to Grow it Nobody would have to worry about getting Laced weed. Marijuana Overdose is not possible because no Human Being can Consume in anyway shape or form 1 Half Ton of Marijuana in 1 sitting. If you need someone to Study on, I Proudly Volunteer. I have used Marijuana since I was 10 years old. It has not slowed down my growth processes what so ever or caused me to get bad grades, do bad in school or use other drugs. Cannabis users who claim Marijuana led them to other drugs are pulling your' chain. They chose the other drugs themselves and when they got caught they used Marijuana as an excuse.

45. Almost always use an o-pen vaporizer....amazing product!

46. Although i have cut down my use of Cannabis, when i was smoking every day I had severe anxiety issues, paranoia, severe social anxiety and depression. I found it very hard to cut down my use but now i have, i smoke around once a week and feel 100% better! As a regular user for 10 years i would never condemn the recreational use of Cannabis but i do not think it is healthy to to smoke it regularly (ie every day) hope this helps :)

47. Although I've had some anxiety lately, the issues are related to my marriage and neither my wife nor I currently use cannabis. When you ask is it addictive, I think anything that floods

your neuroreceptors can cause alternations in the number and sensitivity of those receptors. But do I think someone can become physically dependent on cannabis? No. I think you can get into a rut of inactivity and indulgence which is deleterious to a healthy life, but this can happen with video games or football watching.

48. Although some things I have checked would appear contradictory , i.e - selecting more motivation and less motivation on the same question , but this is because the effects vary based on what I'm smoking and it's thc/cbd ratio cannabis higher in thc makes me want to dance around ,do housework etc.... Higher cbd's tend to give me that feeling of being glued to the sofa. But also a greater sense of relaxation and relief from stress. Both have their places depending on the situation

49. Although when I was going I used marijuana as a recreational drug, things have changed for me. I have chronic pain from degenerative arthritis and fibromyalgia. I find smoking or vaporizing marihuana two or three times a day relieves my pain to acceptable levels, allows me to function, and causes much fewer side effects than the opiates and other pills they try to prescribe to me. I used to take 40 mg a day of opiates until two years ago...I tapered off all pills and began a self-administered regimen of marijuana. I function better, have less agitation, and get better sleep.

50. Anecdotally extremely useful for PTSD-based anxiety, sleep issues (night terrors) and social issues caused by anger

51. Any substance can be addicting, but given the established

scientific understanding of how cannabinoids interact with the body, I believe cannabis to be healthy, and I use it not only for recreational value, but also to prevent future ailments.

52. As a mother of 3 I used marijuana to alleviate symptoms of anxiety/depression/pain. I firmly believe that treating my issues with prescription drugs(as in past) was detrimental to my physical health. Smoking enables me to care for my family with enthusiasm and laughter. Also. Not mentioned in survey was benefits during PMS and PPMD. helps enormously with cramps and irritability.

53. As a public service, public should be informed of the healthiest to most harmful ways of consuming it

54. As a recreational user, I consider cannabis enhances quality of life.

55. As far as addiction goes, I had a difficult time saying just yes or no to whether or not cannabis is addictive. It is not addictive as to where I just need it. I'm addicted to playing video games like I am to consuming cannabis. I play every day, but I don't need to play them to be happy. Video games are an enhancement to life, not life itself. (You can see where I'm going with this.) My body does not react poorly at all when stopping or reducing cannabis intake.

56. asked if Cannabis is addictive. Not really sure how to answer. I think it is, but isn't if that make sense. I have smoked daily for over 6 years now, It helps with my sleep apnea and Ulcerative Colitis/ Crohn's. If I don't have any for a day or two I'm ok. Im not going out to steal or rob money to get it. I'm a functioning

smoker as are most of my friends. I'm not missing house payments or paying bills to get my fix. I think that if Cannabis was legalized and taxed it would help create jobs and help reduce national debt. And if you look at the fact that more people die each year from Alcohol related accidents it would seem to make sense to legalize weed and make Alcohol illegal. But due to the large corporations and lawyers that will never happen. Good luck with your survey

57. At 19 I went to rehab for drugs and alcohol. I went to AA for about 10 years. I stayed sober for about 18. I decided to use Cannabis to help relax after work and it's one of the best decisions of my life. It has improved the quality of my life significantly. I'm happier and I feel more tuned into the universe (which is an extremely silly, stoner thing to say, but this is anonymous). Good luck with the research!

58. Be excellent to one another, and party on

59. before I ever tried cannabis I had somewhat of a 'Short fuse' and would let little things get to me. After my First use that changed dramatically. I now rarely get upset at anything! I am not sure why that would be an effect, maybe something to do with THC interactions in the frontal lobe??

60. before i found cannabis for my stomach/gut issues, i had been completely debilitated by my conditions and was forced to withdraw from school to seek treatment. Because of cannabis, I have a life again, and have re-enrolled in school full time and pulled a 3.78 GPA over the last year. Cannabis has truly changed my life.

61. Before I had medical cannabis, my life was a painful existence. I was on a lot of prescriptions (20 different types) that really didn't help with the pain, nausea, or muscle spasm and kept me very tired/drowsy. my memory barely worked if at all. some of the prescriptions were for side effects of my main prescriptions, but they had side effects of there own. I was in college and a young mother at the time which made it harder for me to do the thing things I needed to do. I found my compassionate doctor through a friend, who thought medical cannabis would help me . I was desperate to get my life back and to be able to remember anything more then a few seconds. So I tried medical cannabis for the first time in my life after getting my first medical cannabis patient card. I was able to eat and keep the food down, I was able to sleep, my nightmares mostly left, my body stopped jerking, and my migraine finally left after 2 years of suffering within minutes. I gained weight which was good since I was 90lbs and dropping before medical cannabis. that's roughly 40 lbs under weight for me. Within 6 months after starting medical cannabis, I went from 20 Rx pills to 1. I could think clearly once again and remember what I had learned in class and my kids when they were little. One of my conditions is PTSD, medical cannabis has helped me greatly. not just with consuming it, but growing it. In my state you can grow your own or have a grower. In short medical cannabis didn't only give me back my life, it gave me back the quality of life.

62. Before my wreck, I smoked to get high. That was the only reason. Since my wreck, I no longer enjoy the getting high part of smoking. I look for more CBD?CBN concentrates for daytime use to be able to be mobile. I will occaisionally use a higher THC content to aid in sleeping, but do worry about

being harrassed for driving under the influence the next day or week. My wife is also a patient, and we are able to grow our own until next August. At that time, we will lose our growing rights since there is a dispensary within 25 miles of our residence.

63. Before trying cannabis I was struggling and it wasn't easy to get a prescription. I finally decided to try cannabis over other stuff. I now feel alive and normal.

64. Before using cannabis, I was unable to sleep because of pain from spinal stenosis. The marijuana capsules which I make have now replaced all pain and sleep medication.

65. Begin in 1930s home remedies for folks in the midwest. Examine the correlation of dosing cbd at 10 mg with 100 mg thc.

66. Beleive it is better and safer than pharmaceuticals.

67. Best for depression, pain nausea and insomnia

68. Better medicine than any pain pills

69. Both medical and recreational use of cannabis needs to be examined in exactly this fashion, and I'm glad I was able to participate. The more information that can be gained, the better.

70. By using my vaporizer, I use less marijuana more effectively with fewer side effects.

71. Caffeine, nicotine, and tobacco are all drugs that are socially

acceptable. I don't see how cannabis has gotten such a bad reputation. In my opinion I can't have worse consequences than the legal drugs and can't be abused worse.

72. can add this is why I can get out of bed without my medication of Canada's I would not be able to get out of bed and it would be costing this government almost $10,000 a month to give me medication I now grow my own medicine please do not take my rights too protect my own medication the pharmaceutical companies are making money the government is saving money I'm trying to help myself become better please do not take those rights from me

73. Canabis has improved my life and my well-being.

74. Cannabis adds a beautiful quality to my life. That being said it can be misused and begin having negative effects as well. Just like alcohol, some people just don't handle their smoke well :)

75. Cannabis adds to the overall quality of my life. I wish I could have safer access to it in Tennessee.

76. Cannabis allowed me to quit using most narcotics for pain. Also don't need anti depressants anymore.

77. Cannabis also excellent remedy for insomnia. I formerly used ambien almost every night. Now I only use it 1-2 times per month. I've also lost almost 40 pound over the past year (healthy rate, not a 'crash' diet). I use cannabis instead of unhealthy food choices (munchies notwithstanding).

78. Cannabis and CBD tinctures provide me with the necessary

level of relief that conventional medicine has not been able to provide.

79. cannabis and its use should be studied very seriously

80. Cannabis can be abused just as any other material item can be abused. Alcohol, cocaine, prescription drugs, and even other items like food can be abused by people. But it's up to the user to make responsible decisions when using the substance. To know when to stop (just like when drinking alcohol), know when too much is too much (just like alcohol), when you aren't suitable to drive when using (just like alcohol), etc.

81. Cannabis can be disruptive in a psychological sense, but if you keep up to date of what your friends and family thinks about you use of Cannabis. Put extra attention to people that tell you that you have changed because of Cannabis. It could be a problem

82. cannabis can be fun but it isnt always for everyone

83. Cannabis can be psychologically addictive, as in habit forming, but not physically addictive, as in withdraw symptoms.

84. Cannabis can be very useful but I believe that it should NOT be marketed as a miracle cure-all to everyone due its side effects. I was suckered into thinking cannabis would improve my life but it led to large amounts of anxiety and lowered productivity. I kept smoking thinking that cannabis was helping me, but in reality it was only hurting me.

85. Cannabis can help M.S users

86. Cannabis changed my life completely for better.

87. Cannabis changes my train of thought and allows me to view events/people from different and varying perspectives. It makes me more analytical, asking 'Why'

88. Cannabis contains beneficial molecules and also intoxicates. This duality causes trouble for people's minds. Couple this trouble with a successful propaganda campaign, and cannabis becomes infamous.

89. cannabis cured my Hep C and everything else... I no longer take any medications of any kind .. after 30 years this is a miracle .my thyroid is normal.

90. Cannabis cures cancer.

91. Cannabis cures cancer. Research by qualified people (that's you!) will save millions of lives. I have lost loved ones, please continue your work

92. Cannabis distracts me from pain.

93. Cannabis does not 'cure' diseases. I am pissed that so many people believe they need it for medical reasons. Many people are acting fraudulently. others are suckered in and now they think they are 'sick' and that pot is the 'cure.' I am tired of people saying they need it for an off-list condition like anxiety. I'm glad that it's now legal in WA. This will keep the jokers from the medical cases. Maybe now we can get some decent medical research done without people using recreationally feeling the need (for fear of the law) to claim medical need and

muddy up the water on its uses.

94. Cannabis doesn't seem chemically addictive but can be psychologically. I feel like it clears my lungs from asthmatic tendencies and sort of opens them up and so I smoke after cigarettes in order to leave them more open or cigarettes after big hits of concentrates so that I cough less. At this point my cigarette habit is too heavy (pack a day) so I feel like it doesn't work anymore but I feel like something about the thc ingestion helps clear/heal/protect lungs from the cigs which was sort of supported by some studies showing that smoking cannabis with tobacco lowered tobacco smokers cancer rates

95. Cannabis gives me a primarily negative experience, (paranoia, depression, anxiety, and slight nausea). It was a positive experience for the first few years of using marijuana (creativity, motivation, positive social interaction), but that changed around 4 years ago when I was 17 for no apparent reason and has never become positive again. I revisit it once or twice a year for introspection and to check in with myself mentally and emotionally, as it brings to light things that are bothering me that I may need to work on.

96. Cannabis had been extremely effective in my life and has caused no negative consequences throughout use history. Much safer than alcohol

97. cannabis has a large variety of medical effects. CBD itself has the ability to inhibit cancer cells. Aswell as many of the cannabinoids in cannabis, Many cases of brain tumors and cancer tumors in the lungs, prostate and kidneys have been sent into remission and even been CURED, by cannabis OIL.

which is mainly a oil consisting of high amounts of CBD, and low amounts of THC.

98. Cannabis has a variety of medicinal uses and many people choose it as a safer form of medication for a variety of ailments, such as pain relief or to treat depression. It can help people with appetite problems and forms of Cannabis exist with no psychoactive ingredients to use purely for medicating. I believe Cannabis is an overall safer substance for both medicine and recreational use for adults. I do not think the Government should decide what people can and cannot ingest as autonomous adults.

99. Cannabis has a very large stigma to overcome. I do believe it to be medicine for me. A medicine I can feel good about, in plant form, that heals me. I also believe it to be addictive. Lots of things are addictive in life. Here are a few of my addictions: baths, reading before bed, meditation in the morning, chocolate, natural spring water from the Lynnwood public well, Holy Basil, Cannabis, Black Pepper, Sole, Tangerines, and Honey. Everything in moderation. It is a life lesson. And for each person that will be a highly individualized process. Know why you use it. Honor the spirit of it. And enjoy the plant.

100. Cannabis has always been portrayed as an evil, addictive drug, compared to much harder drugs. But the truth of it is Cannabis has been so helpful and brought so much good for so many people. It can relieve symptoms of cancer patients, or it can help a stressed out individual relax after a long day at work. The shaming and misconception marijuana has is damaging to our society in many ways. People are jailed for absurd periods of time for marijuana related offenses. When in reality, alcohol

(a legal substance) is significantly worse for you than Cannabis. Yet marijuana users are discriminated and profiled against, to a very unsettling point. Everyone whom I know that has come into contact with Cannabis could not say anything bad about it. The reality of Cannabis, for recreational or medical use, is it truly does help people with very little repercussions. This plant can be a game changing economy booster, reduce crime, and help thousands of more people- if only it were legal in every aspect of the law. Maybe someday that will change.

101. Cannabis has been a Godsend to me as I suffer from anxiety and panic attacks, as well as severe migraines.

102. Cannabis has been a life saver for me in pain management and appetite enhancement.

103. Cannabis has been a much more effective and ultimately rewarding way for me to self-medicate for bipolar disorder. There is a definite balance for me - if I smoke too much I'll get anxiety and paranoia, but when I smoke it in moderation I find that my quality of life improves. I don't sweat the small stuff, I prioritize and make lists to keep myself organized, it really keeps me in check and it's something I really believe can help certain people with mood disorders and mental health issues if used in an unstigmatized, controlled environment. It's a social thing, I've made many great friends through cannabis. It bonded my siblings and I together despite our age and other differences.

104. Cannabis has been a saviour to me since i was diagnosed with crohns. Nothing else touched the pain im in. Its the only thing thats returned my appetite and reduced my nausea. I find it a

crime that its not legal for medical use in my country.

105. Cannabis has been an important adjunct and sometimes replacement for prescription medications. While it does not eliminate my symptoms it makes them more bearable and really helps to keep my mind positive. I believe everyone deserves the right and freedom to choose what they put in their body especially in regards to medication.

106. Cannabis has been an increasingly important part of my life. While I have used it recreationally since 17, it became my only medication 10 years ago just in time to save my life from a deepening and dangerous major depression. It has been key in rehabilitating my life and finding purpose again. I have never been healthier or happier, than I am with cannanbis consumption at reasonable levels.

107. Cannabis has been highly instrumental in resolving long term chronic pain, allowing me to live a pain-free life and effectively run my own business.

108. Cannabis has been in usage for thousands of years with no deaths.

109. Cannabis has changed my life. I was out of shape, depressed and a fairly miserable person prior to starting use. Since becoming a regular user, my life has improved dramatically. I started doing hot yoga 4-5 days a week, am in school getting better grades than I ever did before with more drive to do well. I love it.

110. Cannabis has greatly diminished my menopausal symtoms.

Ambian, which I used for insomnia issues, left me feeling 'strange'. I also had problems w/ Welbutrin. I take one , 500mg cannabis Oil capsule before bed and get a restful nights sleep with NO side effects the next day. It also gives me relief from my arthritis pain.

111. Cannabis has greatly enhanced my quality of life. It is, if nothing else, preventative medicine and should be used as such by more individuals. We all have an endocannabinoid system and THC receptors in our brains. Why else would we have those if we weren't meant to use this wonderful, amazing plant!

112. Cannabis has helped me calm my anxiety and depression a lot. It's only addictive in that it's a lot more fun to be high than it is to be sad.

113. Cannabis has helped me control depression & I am healing. Cannabis consumption is a spiritual practice for me& calms me. I am now learning to be more productive with it & my medical marijuana dispensary is helping me to find the right cannabis flower, a good match that will keep me productive and cheerful.

114. Cannabis has helped me greatly in my life with pain & anxiety. While I FULLY support medical use, it feels as though recreational use or use 'because it's fun' (like alcohol) is taboo. I suffer from chronic pain with a pinched nerve and it helps so much to use cannabis, but I also enjoy using it recreationally with friends or just for the fun of it. It calms me down, helps me focus and I feel good.

115. Cannabis has helped me immensely in the long term

management of crohn's disease, as well as depression and anxiety. Using it daily has greatly increased my quality of life.

116. Cannabis has helped me so much.

117. Cannabis has helped me tremendously since I began inhaling in 2009. I do not use it for pain, but rather for spiritual reasons that helps me assess my life and my internal emotions. Cannabis helps me feel more empathy towards my friends and family, I become more creative in my conversations and open to how I feel. I strongly believe it should be legalized world wide because it can and will help many people out there -- both in terms of physical and psychological. It's truly a wonderful herb of this world that should be used by as many as possible.

118. Cannabis has improved my life and has allowed me to manage my depression and anxiety with a natural substance.

119. Cannabis has improved my life greatly allowing me to drop my vicoden prescription by half. Cannabis also has improved my marriage allowing me and the wife to relax better after the kids go to bed, without the obvious bad side effects of alcohol.

120. Cannabis has improved my quality of life immeasurably. It has helped me cope with issues in my life, relieved my ibs symptoms, and helped with pain management.

121. Cannabis has improved my quality of life physically, & mentally.

122. Cannabis has many positive medical and recreational attributes, some which are striven for by synthetic drugs, and when properly used poses significantly less harm to the user than prescription drugs.

123. Cannabis has played a 100% positive role in my life. My only problem is when I forget to use it. I used to be a coffee addict, and my life was a wreck. Switching to just weed I'm finding love of life again, not to mention sleep.

124. Cannabis has proved useful in all areas of my life. Recreationally, medically and academically. Medically I use it for pain management, muscle fatigue, general fatigue and motivation, anger and irritability, stress, anxiety, depression, poor appetite, muscle spasms, increased focus and concentration, and general increased mood. Recreationally I use it to reduce worry and stress, sleep better, eat regularly. I use it to relax and not worry about school or small arguments in relationships. Spiritually I used it to slow down, connect with the world around me, appreciate people, exercise, relax and find calm stillness and peace. Academically I use it open my mind towards higher thought, to think out of the box, organize and research.

125. cannabis has saved my life by allowing me to get off soo many pharmaceuticals & live a pain free musclw spasm free life

126. Cannabis has started giving me panic attacks that last about 20 hours, after only taking two or three hits. My heart races, my neck feels hot, and everything spins and I get shaky and scared. I know this is atypical, but my mom had the same symptoms from use when she was my age. It didn't used to happen, I smoked for about a year before anything bad happened, but now it's horrible and I've stopped using it altogether.

127. Cannabis helped me through depression in my first year of university while I was in residence. It is where I first started smoking heavily and instead of getting wasted off of alcohol all

the time like it was popular to do, I stayed lifted and dove into art and music and film with other like minded individuals. I could have gone the other way I guess. I used it to cope and I maybe it is a crutch, but I am happy that I refused pharmaceutical prescriptions from doctors. I think pills would have numbed me from the journey that I needed to take in order to start feeling better. Cannabis helped me realize my dreams and now I am working to achieve them. I wish I didn't face the stigma of being a pot head, I want to working with children as a teacher but I am afraid that other adults will think less of me because I smoke it recreationally and medicinally. Cannabis has made me a better person.

128. Cannabis helped me to stop the prescription pain killers I took for nearly ten years.

129. cannabis helps me like no other drug out there while high i feel happy im interested in talking to others it helps me sleep it helps with bad things going on around me it blocks out bad emotions and negative thoughts, there's no headache or sickness its just a shame i have to buy from dodgey dealers i'd rather buy from a respected company like the local store or dispensary if it were to be legalized then id know what am smoking is safe and wouldnt be getting robbed all the time. see thats what some dealers do they take your money and you never get the weed or they mix it with other stuff to weigh it down id rather pay the government TAX than go to a street dealer it be much safer.

130. Cannabis helps me sleep well and is a fun recreational drug. When I use regularly I sleep better, but often my appetite is small unless I toke. When 'quitting' or stopping, diarrhea is the worse symptom and lasts for about 4 to 5 days. All things

considered, the joy and benefit I get from using cannabis vastly outweighs the negative things.

131. Cannabis helps me to feel fully present in the moment and in my body, strengthening my senses. At the same time, it brings me into a dream world and stimulates my imagination and creativity. I view it as an ally. I do not depend on it, but it enriches my life.

132. Cannabis improves my ability to endure hardship.

133. Cannabis improves the quality of life for so many people. It has been used for thousands of years and only in the last hundred years has it been considered anything but helpful. We need to stop prohibition if the human race is to move on to a better future. Hemp and Cannabis hold the key to our future and without them we will not last long on this planet.

134. Cannabis in itself is not addictive, however it can be used as a crutch to reduce anxiety and pain. This creates a mental dependency. I could quit smoking immediately and not see any adverse effects, however It has become the norm in my life to smoke and this is hard to cvercome.

135. Cannabis in many ways has improved my quality of life dramatically. Sleep apnea and anxiety often impaired my ability to be myself and thrive. I used Cannabis in high school strictly recreational though after five years (4 in the USMC) I began using for medicinal purposes. After using I was so focused and relaxed that I ended up starting my own business and was able to change many life habits for the better. For myself cannabis has been a wonderful thing. Although I do have concerns

about prolonged exposure to its smoke. I know of one study done by Columbia University that did not report to positively about its affects on the lungs in comparison to tobacco. I also did a capstone research project on marijuana for my undergrad degree. If you are interested I can send over.

136. Cannabis instantly eases my pain, anxiety, nausea, and fatigue. If i set an intention before I take cannabis, I find it works better.

137. Cannabis is a Huge benefit to me.

138. Cannabis is a beautiful mind opening herb that gives one perspective and makes you more empathetic. It's affect on music is life-changing. That being said, there is a real possibility of over-use and one should always be able to take a step back and assess one's use

139. Cannabis is a great addition to any fungus foray!

140. Cannabis is a great substance when used in moderation. It is by no means a 'miracle drug,'but it is also by no means a detrimental drug. It is very therapeutic as well as not detrimental to the body in any way. It is psychologically addictive, however, and I can personally vouch for that. Cannabis does not hurt anybody and the chances of someone committing a violent crime while solely under the effects of cannabis are extremely low. It should be legalized and regulated like alcohol and tobacco and we should just move on.

141. Cannabis is a life saver. It is a shame that the current legal status makes patients into criminals. I experience exceptional relief of inflammation in my body. A reduction in ocular pressure has been noted by my ophthalmologist as well.

142. Cannabis is a MUCH cheaper alternative to chronic pain than the prescription medications (all with side effects) and more easily obtainable, especially to those who cannot afford or fall between the cracks with health insurance!

143. Cannabis is a natural substance provided by Earth that should be harnessed by human beings to help better the world.

144. Cannabis is a nutriceutical, a food that works like a drug. It directly influences the Endocannabinoid System which runs mammal physiology. There is no more beneficial her or plant on the planet. It is or can be made into food, fuel, medicine, clothing, packaging, rope, plastic, and building materials.

145. Cannabis is a plant not a drug. Don't let the government warp your mind! We are the people!

146. Cannabis is a plant...a safe, natural, herbal medicine, that heals!

147. cannabis is a strong and beautiful medicine. im a big fan.

148. Cannabis is a super healthy alternative to using over the counter pain medications or sleep aids.

149. Cannabis is a teacher. It will teach a person to achieve states of being that are healthy and happy. If one pays attention to the lessons, one uses less. If one becomes ill, it will help the body to heal. As the body heals one uses less, if one pays attention. It taught me not to use even small amounts of alcohol, showed me how debilitating alcohol is to the cells of the body. The munchies are mostly an attempt by the body to make one aware of dehydration. Drinking water will diminish the munchies

if one is not hungry. Best to take cannabis when not hungry. Using small amounts will not decrease one's ability to operate a vehicle, but one ought not be high enough to have a sense of time alteration when one drives. A little use can make one more relaxed and therefore a better driver, less hurried and more in tune with the experience of being in the moment.

150. Cannabis is a valuable medicine which helps me manage a birth defect called NPS (Nail-Patella Syndrome).

151. Cannabis is addictive, but it's not like cigarettes or alcohol. Cannabis addiction is an addiction to a lifestyle of laziness. Although it does not necessarily impact your motivation, it is very easy to just sit on your couch and smoke pot all day. You won't get in any fights, you won't beat your wife; but you won't be looking for a job either.

152. Cannabis is an amazing plant that nature has provided for us, humans, to enjoy. Cannabis has many more positive aspects than negative. I have the utmost respect for cannabis and I use it in moderation.

153. Cannabis is an amazing plant. It helps tremendously with my depression, anxiety, amnesia, and anger issues. It also keeps me from smoking 60 cigarettes a day and it helps prevent me from drinking myself into an early grave. Cannabis also calmed me down and allowed me to attend mainstream school at thirteen years old, to earn eleven GCSE grades after only three years of education. Cannabis sharpens my mind and makes me human. Thank you, Cannabis.

154. Cannabis is an excellent medicinal tool that helps many all

around the world, and should be taken out of schedule 1 and made more readily available for study and use.

155. Cannabis is an herb that heals. There are so many ways to use it for home health, far beyond an altered state. This comes in the form of sprays and oils for skin, skin care, hair care, juicing and the like. I understand that the leaves can also be eaten raw for significant health benefits. Bastyr is a wonderful organization that has the ability to look outside of the pharmacy for natural and organic healing. It would be a blessing to see Bastyr research and develop outcomes that would be well respected and received within the community, and help individuals on their path to better wellness. Thank you.

156. Cannabis is an untapped resource

157. Cannabis is balm for the troubled, medicine for those in pain, a social and recreational drug that never leads to violence, can be grown anywhere, and is safe except for rare respiratory conditions. I had not known of its medicinal qualities until recently, having been a recreational user, but knew of some mild sleep and appetite problems being solved. Cannabis, when used by experienced people, can be a wonderful enhancement for sexual activity, food and drink, visually stimulating experiences such as theatre or movies, and a great aid for relaxed communication. Music takes on new meaning and nuance when one uses Cannabis.I have used it since my youth, hroughout my military service, and all through my working life without ill effect. I understand the drug, and so use it appropriately and in the right social setting. It is not for everyone, and I admit to some mild, transient paranoia when I've used unexpectedly potent varieties, but these feelings always subside.

158. Cannabis is different for everyone. There are so many different strains of marijuana that affect people differently, so in a way its quite difficult to place cannabis on a spectrum ranging from 'good' or 'bad'. Sometimes it may make you paranoid, other times you are relaxed and content. It really depends. Regardless, I believe marijuana to be useful as a plant itself rather than a drug; hemp has been used in many cultures for hundreds and hundreds of years as a resource.

159. Cannabis is food

160. Cannabis is good for the soul

161. Cannabis is great for expanding the mind, feeling connected to other people and the universe. God's love can befelt through cannabis.

162. Cannabis is Great!

163. Cannabis is habitual, but far from addictive. It also serves as a much safer alternative to alcohol

164. Cannabis is healing my Stroke brain. I'm very open to helping with the proper doze of cannabis. My name is xxxxxxxxx please feel free to contact me xxx-xxx-xxxx xxxxxxx@xxxx.com I really want to help!

165. Cannabis is illegal in England so I have no way of selecting what kind of strain to smoke. I just have to buy what's for sale. This is why some of the short-term effects I have stated may seem contradictory as different strains have different side effects and I am unable to obtain a consistent product. Regarding alcohol

consumption, I put 3 drinks a day. I may not drink everyday, but if I do go out for a drink maybe once or twice in the week then 3 is a good average. Intake may increase at weekends.

166. cannabis is illegal in my country

167. Cannabis is illegally persecuted. you cannot have laws against nature. it's a plant FFS. but you knew that :)

168. Cannabis is just a plant, no different then any other and should NOT be ILLEGAL, its horrible, some of the first american laws were that farmers had to grow Hemp, and could pay there tax's with it, if not for human consumption then at least as a product that has more then 5000 known use's and make oil, paper, rope, cloths and more all out of cannabis.

169. Cannabis is like alot like most substances. Its effects are varied by user and situation. A lazy person will be lazy with or without cannabis. A dependent person will be dependent on whatever there into at the moment. And cannabis is the best option.

170. Cannabis is like anything, too much is usually not good but when used in moderation it is a really powerful and safe substance. I trust my source/grower and have also grown my own so I couldn't answer your question about selecting my cannabis, in that case I try what people give me and there is a difference in how the different strains make you feel. I prefer ones that give me energy and motivation since I never have a problem sleeping when I want to. It is a very social thing and I enjoy smoking with my friends or being around people who smoke cannabis. I am not much of a drinker and could never handle tobacco so it is nice to have a social substance

that I can tolerate and even enjoy. Like most things I think it is important for people to take a break from time to time to really know what purpose it is serving in their life. I have never had a problem stopping or abstaining for days/weeks or months at a time. A very sacred plant, so happy it is being looked at in a more positive way.... I feel the paranoia partially stems from the fact that people go to jail for just having a joint. I think legalization is key to removing a lot of the paranoia that people get when they try it. Thanks!

171. cannabis is medicine

172. CANNABIS IS MEDICINE AND A SUPER NICE WAY TO FIND MY DEEPEST THOUGHTS AND AN SPIRITUAL EXPERIENCE

173. Cannabis is Medicine!

174. Cannabis is more complicated than describing the plant with only one effect. The fact you ask about strains is good. Obviously the use of cannabis is much safer than alcohol for the individual and society as a whole.

175. cannabis is natural plant given to us by nature, and it's benefits are endless.

176. Cannabis is not a drug. Not anymore than tobacco or alcohol. Its been outlawed so rich men could get richer. It needs to be legalised. Free the weed.

177. Cannabis is not a harmful substance or dangerous. And it's not for everybody.

178. cannabis is not at all physically addictive. alcohol, caffeine, nicotine (w/o meditation) heroin, etc. definitely are. from a recreational perspective cannabis can be mentally addicitve, like any over indulgence, from ice cream to watching tv. i consider safe access to this special plant a profound blessing.

179. Cannabis is not really distributed here as medication except in exceptional circumstances. As such, it distorts some of the answers above- when I can find the right kind, the negative symptoms like anxiety, depression, and munchies go away. I don't always have access to quality product, and when I do I don't have access to the percentages of CBD etc. I find it immensely helpful for sleeping on especially anxious nights. It also helps when I am depressed (I was on medication, but stopped under doctor recommendations), because it lightens my mood. I think it's generally harmless. Also, it would be interesting to put a comment section under the 'Is cannabis addictive' section. I think you would get some very interesting replies. I think, for myself, it can be something you grow mentally reliant on as a comforting thing, but not physically addicted to. Cheers and good luck with the study!

180. Cannabis is only addictive if you let it be.

181. Cannabis is only addictive in such A way that video games or anything enjoyable is. You like it you want to do more. But I'm not dependent just a habitual user with no desire to stop use

182. Cannabis is plainly not meant to be Schedule I, it's therapeutic uses are vast.

183. Cannabis is safe and effective, time tested and true unlike all

these drugs the FDA throws at us and recalls a moment later due to safety issues. I'll stick with what works for me, what I know is right and true no matter what the law says, though it breaks my heart I would be considered a 'criminal'. The only 'crime' I am committing would, theoretically, be against myself which is no ones issue but my own.

184. Cannabis is something that is subjective to everyone, no one has the same experience, even when you begin to start taking it you may not enjoy it however after 2 weeks when your mental barriers are broken you can begin to enjoy it as is based on a recent experiment I did, it suggests there must be mental and physical adaptation to cannabis perhaps the cannabinidol system need to be activated before accepted into the body

185. Cannabis is tha healing of tha Nation...legalise it everywhere in tha world.

186. Cannabis is the best thing out there for everything.Not a drug--its a plant--in 1940-it was legal--and used then for medicine. You do not over dose--it helps for cancer RSO--and is a heck of alot safer than meth-heroine-crack--AND ALCOHOL

187. Cannabis is the most useful plant on this planet.

188. Cannabis is the only thing that has been effective for severe migraines due to cancer treatment. It was an amazing apetite stimulant during chemotherapy - without it, I gagged on food, and when I smoked food tasted so much better and I did not gag. I have had a few bad experiences with edibles and flowers that made me paranoid/anxious, but have experimented and found strains that do not cause this. I checked off 'edibles' but

actually prefer sublingual delivery (lollipops, hard candies).

189. Cannabis is the only thing that relieves my nausea and pain without further damaging my liver (I have compromised liver function due to Hepatitis C). It is also the only thing that relives my gut pain (I've had three intestinal surgeries since 2009) without further damaging my liver and impairing my motor functions, as opiate narcotics do.

190. Cannabis is the only thing that will rid me of nausea and stomach cramps during menstruation or the flu!

191. Cannabis is very good at reducing my chronic pain from diabetic neuropathy. I am on so many other medications for other health conditions like high blood pressure, high blood fats, thyroid, etc. I like how fast it works and how I can adjust the amount. Pain or not it sure feels good!

192. Cannabis is wonderful for so many reasons. I've never seen it ruin a life, and it certainly hasn't mine.

193. Cannabis kills cancer, I smoked tobacco for 25 years, now I smoke cannabis to ward off lung cancer

194. Cannabis makes life a higher quality. (Lol) it makes you feel motivated and hopeful about the future, it helps you find the good things in life, it let's you be able to laugh like you've never laughed before. Cannabis is the plant of life.

195. Cannabis needs to be legal. Its the alcohol and prescription drugs that need to be looked at. They are the damaging drugs. Cannabis is a plant, a vegetable a way of life. Let's get healthy!!!

196. Cannabis oil kills cancer

197. Cannabis reacts differently with everyone. I personally think it should be legal it causes little harm is done and does not kill anyone, as to the leagal drug alcohol. I don't think it affects the driving in fact I think itmakes me more aware of my surroundings and how I'm driving and last cannibis makes me as a person feel good about my self. Helps me not fall under the pressures of what the media wants. But helps me see the beautiful curvy wemon of the world. And help me look passed all that to who someone really is.

198. Cannabis saves lives!

199. Cannabis saves lives!

200. Cannabis should be legal across the board!

201. Cannabis should be legal to any consenting adult over the age of 21.

202. Cannabis should be legal....I smoke it regardless but I think with alcohol being legal, and it's much worst, that cannabis should be legal, it would calm a lot of people down and I believe it is much less dangerous them alcohol.

203. Cannabis should be viewed as a health and wellness product, not an intoxicant.

204. Cannabis should been legalized both recreational and medial!!!!

205. Cannabis should not be illegal.

206. Cannabis should not be illegal.. God grew it I'm gonna smoke it!

207. Cannabis sometimes help me to relax, I think it is very peaceful, and if anything should be illegal it's alcohol. Leagize it!

208. Cannabis tends to enhance most things in my life, it's very multi-purpose. I tend to find it more pleasant using a small amount at a time. Any anxiety I experience is due to prohibition (fear of being caught, mainly by parents but police to a small extent). It tends to help me to live in the moment and appreciate life. It reinforces what is important to me (eg. music, art, nature, wellbeing, the moment), which helps me to enjoy life as much as possible. It also enhances my appreciation and doing of such things. More long term, cannabis (and other psychedelic drugs, particularly LSA and MDMA) have helped me to become closer to myself and be more honest with myself. It's difficult to explain in writing, but they have had a huge impact on my life, which has been mainly positive. I find the positives tend to hugely outweigh the negatives (negatives including fear of being caught and social anxiety)

209. Cannabis unlocks parts of my consciousness that I never knew existed I can almost live the future through extreme cannabis use and it has exposed my mind to the horrible atrocities happening across the world and the freedoms and liberties being taken away from me in my own country.

210. Cannabis usage varies widely from person to person.

211. Cannabis, as with any other mind altering substance should be used responsibly and in moderation. A 'newbie' should

approach this substance dose by dose, until the individual figures out his/her tolerance level and what It does for them, be it positive or negative.

212. Cannabis, for me, isn't a fixed dose, fixed response medication. As a result, my usage patterns aren't typically consistent. I use more when I need more and use less when I need less. In addition, sometimes one effect will be more prominent with a specific strain (terpenoid profile) or with a specific starting emotional state. As a result, the effects listed above do not all occur with any single dosage, but have been experienced occasionally with certain strains and various prior moods. Furthermore, some of the effects listed above are actually effects of my disease itself and are only exacerbated, not caused, by cannabis use - this may be a confounding factor...

213. Cannabis, I believe, is a far safer drug than alcohol.

214. Cannabis, just like any other drug, has both negative and positive effects. I believe that the use of cannabis to treat ailments or for recreation should be completely legal as it is a safer alternative than alcohol. It is a shame that society deems use of cannabis morally corrupting or generally bad. Cannabis is a substance that can be abused just like alcohol can. It is time to take the stigma off and open the world's eyes to the truth. There are more positives than negatives that would result from legalization - either medicinal or recreational.

215. Cannabis, like any entheogen, requires you to have your personal mental health modulated. Walking the line between inspiration and (maybe) madness, I cannot decide if it's better for me to ingest or not. I usually lean toward not partaking. I

think I've been too close a few times to shy away from cannabis...

216. Cannabis, like any legal or illegal drug, has positive/beneficial and negative/destructive uses and the only person who can determine how it affects them is ones self, unless of corse you are infringing on other peoples rights to freedom or safety, then that is clearly destructive and not determined by the user.

217. Cannabis, to me, brings back the child like wonderment that is missing as we become adults. The feeling that anything is possible and that there is adventure left in the world. It brings about the insight and creativity inherent in us all that is so easy to forget amidst the drudgery that society seems to think is so important.

218. Cannibis has been the only thing that has halted the episodes of my trigeminal neuralgia. I've been episode free for 10 months, my other medications never stopped the episodes, only reduced the frequency to about 4-6 times a year. prior to medication, my episodes were roughly 2 to 4 episodes a month. The side affects of the medications were worse than cannibis.

219. Cannibis is less harmful than alcohol or television.

220. CBD rich hemp oil is helping to dampen the pain of my chronic headache brought on by a brainstem stroke. I also enjoy a slight high from crumbling a little hash into my tea, normally in the evening.

221. Changing from pharmaceuticals to cannabis saved my life. It hasn't made it perfect but I will never go back big pharma.

222. Check out the work of DC Donald Epstein he did personal research that showed him that people who use cannabis and psychedelics healed faster than those who didn't.

223. Choosing types did not have a choice for 'whatever I am able to grow'.

224. chronic pain issues (neck, shoulder, hip)

225. College student. With cannabis related criminal record. Simple possession resulting in time served. Moved cross country to finish college.

226. combustion is the main problem.

227. Compliments on a well-designed questionnaire from someone who also does this for a living.

228. Confusion at dispensaries. Most people who work there don't know about medical impacts.

229. consuming medibles is the most effective way to treat chronic pain

230. Correlation between head injury and cannabis use? Good for treating atypical depression. Starting medical use in early twenties avoided developmental issues surrounding adolescent use. Sativex is essentially hash oil. Fills the void created by discontinuing religious belief. Does Cannabis cause HPPD? Objectively safer than alcohol. Psychedelic component can help change behaviors, for better or worse. Reduces or eliminates risk of self harm. Due to anti-inflammatory properties has

good application for many ailments. Pure Cannabinoid oil aka Rick Simpson Oil, can aid in the elimination of topical cancers applied externally. Personally have not experienced panic attacks caused by cannabis. Panic attacks caused by cannabis may be due to sudden intensification of senses with low tolerance.

231. Crippling back pain and arthritis reduced significantly, allowing a more active and productive lifestyle, higher activity level due to reduced body/back pain resulting in a loss of 45 pounds, (260-215). Migraines reduced from 6-10 moderate to severe (emergency room visit/shot in the ass once or twice yearly) a year, down to 1-2 a year (with no ER visits), cholesterol levels reduced, high blood pressure reduced. most recent check-up revealed all improved numbers. Chronic terrifying nightmares reduced to nil. secondary benefit: Oral hygiene improved. Gingivitis reversed due to more brushing to cover up the smell.

232. Curious as to the relationship between usage maturity and perceived impact of use... I.e. how one consumes shifts over time

233. Dependent on strains (ie sativa or indica dominant) I can do school work more effectively. If I smoke indica strains its harder for me to do school work then if I had smoked a sativa strain. With the sativa strains it is easier to see complicated pathways or mechanisms then it is without

234. Depending on the strain it's good for a myriad of things. Fun, relaxation, pain management etc...

235. Depending on the strain of marijuana I use, I can feel either

more creative or less creative, more motivated or less motivated, more social or less social. Some of those answers will likely be contradictory.

236. Device needed to determine how stoned you are, like a breathalyzer.

237. Diagnosed schizoaffective

238. diagnosed with bipolar . and depression, insomnia and anxiety. it helps with everything and I can be safely off my meds with cannabis

239. Different strains can have very different effects on any given user. I've noticed a wide variety of different types of smokers. I am not what you would call a 'functional stoner'. I do not like going to work that way. I prefer to use it as a relaxation after work and after everything that needs to be done for the day is done. However, my husband is the exact opposite. It motivates him. It is the first thing he does in the morning and does not typify the lazy stoner stereotype. I also know people who use it for the severe & debilitating nausea they suffer from on a daily basis. The doctor cannot figure out what is wrong and the medications they prescribe do little to help. Cannabis has been the only thing she has found to allow her to get through her day - go to work, school and deal with family. Otherwise, she would be completely debilitated by this.

240. Different strains have very different effects. Some strains make you feel like you have ADHD and shiny objects distract you, while others give you super in depth focus. Some make everything seem funny, some just make you feel elated. Some

make you sleepy and help with pain reduction (CBD). CBD has fantastic anti-nausea properties. I have social anxiety and CBD edibles or flower with low THC content I 100% feel ok driving with. I have gotten into the car and realized I was probably too stoned to drive, but I think it makes you drive very slow and careful whereas with Alcohol you feel like you're ok to go and you don't compensate. Some give you a heavy weight on your eyes and couch lock for zoning out. There are some strains I keep around just for yard work/cleaning as it just makes it more fun :D

241. Different strands used have a huge effect on my high. I will be more motivated and clear headed or tired and hungry. I believe it alters with the amount of THC in the strand

242. Different types/levels of constituents in marijuana seem to have opposing effects. I can either be more or less anxious. Can also vary with amount smoked. I began using marijuana while also using prescription drugs and alcohol. I now do not consume either and have greatly reduced my marijuana intake as well.

243. Disabled but not handicapped, I'm in year nine of being a GBM survivor, when the diagnosis included a median life expectancy of 16 months. Now predisposed for seizures, I've been waking daily and having my first of 6 or 7 smoking sessions for over 5 1/2 years, after my first post brain surgery seizure. I volunteer in my community, xxxxxxxxxxxxxxxxxxxxxxxxxxxxxxxxxx , walk and play golf in the 80s, where joints are usually followed by a par or better. 185 rounds last year.

244. Disabled Veteran with PTSD.

245. DISCONTINUATION OF USE: I get headaches, but it takes 3 days before I realize the headaches are from running out of cannabis. This is why I say it's not addictive. I have done pills & meth in my youth (more than 15yrs ago) & I knew exactly what I was craving for when I ran out (ie addictive), but w/ cannabis the symptoms somehow seem unrelated to running out. I hope that makes sense.

246. Don't be so interested in my personal information. You do not need my mothers maifen name to know why I smoke pot

247. dont fuck up the market price on it dont over regulate and over tax it. let the little guy get in on the new industry!!

248. Dose size is very important, controlling dose is trickier than most people expect.

249. Driving high is not a problem. All stoners do it everyday. Take away weed DUI laws

250. Driving under cannabis influence differs depending on tolerance. Addictiveness depends on ones mental state (being non-skitzo) and basic willpower. I do not find it hard to quit for a month, however I do not ignore the fact that I have mild side effects from quitting abruptly. Take care.

251. Each high is different. The negative effects noted above result mainly from consuming too much cannabis for one's tolerance level. Tolerance builds, but is reduced with breaks from cannabis.

252. Edible hash oil (sometimes known as 'Rick Simpson oil') seems

to be the most effective form of cannabis for reducing seizures, for me. Vaping and smoking may help with some of the other effects of epilepsy (tics, auras, partial seizures), but they are not nearly as effective as a few drops of hash oil each day for preventing tonic clonic seizures.

253. ENDOCANNABINOID SYSTEM in r bodies,feed that CANNABINOIDS from hemp plant,by juicing,eating the bud,or making the life saving oil from the plant,means healthy n happy,GOD BLESS all of us when something so simple could do so much.

254. Endocannabinoid system is mind blowing

255. Even those using cannabis 'recreationally' are using it medicinally for anti-stress or relaxation purposes. The public should have easy access to cannabis. The distinction made between recreation and medical use is false and synthetic. We should be doing a better job of articulating the importance of healthy medicines and personal involvement with our healthcare.

256. Ever since I first used cannabis, I felt it was something i wanted to have every day. I'm in pharmacy school now, presenting myself as a person who's interested in the science and practice of using cannabis to help people, but I worry it's been a story i tell myself to justify me using cannabis compulsively. I'm taking a more critical look at myself to see how cannabis is affecting my life negatively, and how i can reset my relationship with the drug to one that's in line with my long term goals for my mindset, and for my action plans.

257. Everyone should have access to clean and safe cannabis and should be able to choose formulation. I don't qualify for medical cannabis.

258. Factors in selecting cannabis: can't select, based on what my dealer has. Methods of cannabis use: you forgot about spliffs (cannabis or hash mixed with tobacco) which is very common in Europe. Disregard my reply about puffs, when you smoke a spliff puffs won't apply.

259. Far better than any pain medicine i currently take, helps my mood, makes me upbeat, It's Fantastic

260. Feeling good makes the body heal itself heal. Recreational use is medial use.

261. Fibromuscular dysplasia can be complicated with many symptoms requiring different types of meds. I take none of them thankfully for cannabis.

262. Finding the proper strain for your particular need is the key to reaping benefit from this course of therapy. Sadly I cannot find my strain locally so I am forced to use 4x more of a different 'flavor', which i've been told is the best around.

263. for me it take of all the stress and helps me to forget i have tinintus for a vild

264. For me the most discouraging part of my cannabis use is that it's nearly impossible for me to handle working and having to be around people without the self medication with cannabis I practice, but my use prohibits getting and keeping most jobs in my area (and probably any other area in the country).

265. For me, cannabis is both a recreational substance, as well as a therapeutic wellness product.

266. For me, cannabis provides a life line to a life I wouldn't be able to comfortably without. I suffer from chronic pain and cannabis either improves the pain or allows me to ignore it. I often find myself able to concentrate on what I'm doing rather then just feeling uncomfortable. However, on occasion I find that I become too engrossed in whatever I'm doing and that can be detrimental.

267. For me, moderation is preferable to the more significant amount I used as a young adult. I love mj and live music. Thx for your work.

268. For me, sometimes smoking pot feels like an issue, and sometimes it is just something I enjoy. I have seen other people struggle with anxiety, depression and loss of a sense of control with their use. When I am going through a high-stress time, using can ease temporary anxiety, but increase a stress-cycle. I have mental illness history in my family, but have never been diagnosed myself.

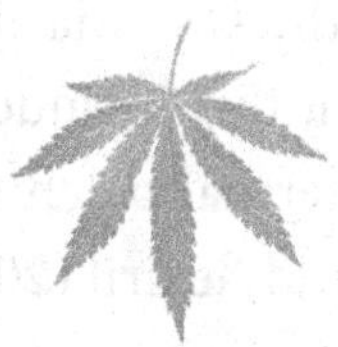

269. For my entire life, I've dealt with pain, digestive, sleep, and social anxiety issues. Sadly, I lived in a state that didn't allow access to MMJ. So instead of getting the treatment that worked best for me, I had to deal with medications that only sort of worked. Then at my worst points of pain/digestive issues, I had to risk arrest just to get low grade medication. This year I moved to WA for non MMJ reasons, and as a bonus got myself a 'card'. Since I've been a MMJ patient my quality of life has improved DRASTICALLY. The pain I used to experience is rarely an issue anymore, I sleep better, I am calmer, and my digestive issues are less frequent. The strange thing is, I only medicate in the evening before I go to bed. Yet the relief I get from MMJ seems to stay with me until the early evening hours. Medical marijuana has been a life improving medication for me, and I hope through honest studies like these, more non-mmj patients will see the benefits.

270. For the past 5 years I have been a chronic pain patient trying nearly anything and everything recommended by doctors. I've seen physical therapists, occupational therapists, mental health professionals, pain management specialists, doctors that deal with chronic pain, etc. I am a former athlete that has been rendered to a fairly sedentary lifestyle since my injury. Marijuana is the only thing that resolves my pain. I've been prescribed nearly every major short term and long term pain reliever available in the US. Marijuana is by far the best thing to eliminate my pain, this includes surpassing the effects of a daily fentanyl transdermal patch (50 mcg/hr) + hydrocodone (up to 60 mgs/day) and flexiril (20mgs/day).

271. For the question 'How freqently [sic] do you use Cannabis?', the answers, in my case, were limiting from a relatable perspective.

I chose 1-4 times a day. It would be good to have the option of 'Once a day' as I only smoke in the evening after I've finished whatever I have to do. Unless 1-4 times a day doesn't mean concurrent hits off a pipe, for example.

272. For those who use it for rec purposes it's does just as much bad as good. I to helps people who use it for health purposes it's great. It does more good than bad, it's a winner in my book

273. Forty years ago it provided an alternative to alcohol. When I was diagnosed with prostate cancer in 2006, cannabis became official medicine, a strong ally against cachexia, pain and PTSD. Not merely 'recreational' (belittling term), but life-supporting. Read the book:www.createspace.com/3454863

274. Free all cannabis users from all prisons!

275. From 1st hand hand experience smoking it while ur your going through some bad times and relying on it can mentally mess you up but its all about will power and how you control it. I used to get really paranoid but now when I smoke I know its the marijuana making me feel that so i calm my self down when I think that but ive heard from people who have beenbto amsterdam and places and they tell me that tue weed there doesn't five u the bad feelings like it does in uk. Now im not to sure if its tye strain or if its mental.

276. From being a recreational smoker to working in the massive pot gardens of northern california I see up close and personal of what not only smoking but absorbing thru your skin does to people. I think yes it is addictive to those that smoke daily but at the same time I believe I could quit cold turkey... But do I want

to no never. I have children and live where it's recreationally legal. Cannabis is a special plant with many properties.

277. From my Experiance using Cannabis as a pain reliever is that it doesn't kill the pain like a opiate but it allows me to deal with the pain in a sense like I forget it's there. I also get the ability if the pain is more intense to take more without worries of ODing. Pairs very well with My Morning Jacket

278. From using it for recreation to medicinal.. I need those cbd's and cbcs! My father was in vietnam, my sister and I both have birth defects.. its the only thing that makes quality of life worth living again. I remember when it was just fun before I hurt my back.. now, its merely a necessity such as toilet paper.. I hope this helps us that aren't mmp yet and your study as well. thank you

279. Full time student, working on BS degree. Reason for choosing Unemployed, AA highest education achieved. Using cannabis as a substitute for alcohol, and other drugs were no because there wasn't ever a need to substitute it. I've chosen to use Cannabis over alcohol before though, if that counts as substituting it?

280. Generally speaking, the Venn diagram of medical vs recreational users has a large overlap, but they are two separate communities with different needs. I fear that the recent Washington legalization and current attempts - despite promises - to regulate mmj along with recreational use will jeopardize vulnerable patients.

281. gods holy plant, best medicine around, never lets me down, END PROHIBITION

282. Good Evening, I hope U and your family are at peace tonight....... as I have never being a drinker, I have inhaled cannabis for many reasons on and off for 40 years. As a product of a broken home at 2yrs and sexually abused as a child, I never received any therapy in my adult life. I began smoking weed when I was 15, tripped on acid 1x at 16 and I tried speed, ludes, coke and I ODed at 18 on PCP. Detoxed for about a year and at 19 became pregnant, cleaned my act up, landed good job in printing took classes. On and off smokin' weed but not a big deal. At 24 I working 2 jobs, 8 hours printing, 5 to 6 hours closing a restaurant daily 6 and 7 days a week. One of my girls turned me on to crank, I believe they call it meth now, I carried on for about 6 months, till the connection ran out and I switched over to coke, it didn't work the same but a nice substitute except at 26 I started smoking it ......I have more I want to say, but I need to give this a break....this is a lot to tell some one I have never met, you may not need all this useless info, it's just that I have been trying to find some one that is doing research in this area, so that I maybe able to contribute my experiences to the study as evidence....if U want, U can contact me at xxxxxxxxx@xxxxxx.com ~Thank You for this opportunity~

283. good luck

284. Good luck and have fun! Also, I prefer to buy from the medical dispensary than the recreational shops because the taxes are crazy high (intended).

285. Good luck with the study!

286. Good question. I appreciate you asking me this. Firstly, I believe that there is an ethical obligation to protect users of cannabis

against criminalisation under common law, which is causing harm, theft or injury; clearly none of these apply to cannabis use. For me, the prohibition of nature seems nonsensical. It is one of the greatest tragedies of modern times that the lives of people and those around them are ruined by being incarcerated for non violent crimes. My health and cannabis use background: I have been using cannabis frequently since the age of 11, and now at the age of 17 I remain incredibly healthy. I eat well; a staple diet of fruits, vegetables and nuts and grains for energy and quality meat once in a while. I believe this is the foundation of my health, as it is giving my body the nutrients it desires to protect itself and thus my great pulmonary health. I do not not formally practice exercise, but I have no difficulty carrying out athletic tasks like sprinting up hills and cycling 20 miles, of which do not make me breathless as may be the case for a heavy tobacco smoker. When I was working in the summer and making a lot of money I was using 2 ounces a week which is the equivalent of 112-168 joints that contain tobacco or 56 blunts containing only cannabis. Now I only smoke a gram a day which is the equivalent of 3 joints. I am aware that cannabis smoke contains carcinogens but I smoke joints as it is my form of luxury. Whenever I don't have any money to buy cannabis, it is never on my mind, I never feel like there is something lacking in my life. But when I do have cannabis, I feel content like I don't need anything else. For this reason cannabis is not a gateway drug, and if I were to buy alcohol (never) or class A drugs (about 3 times a year) I will definitely need cannabis. I am a horticulturist, and in the future I plan on growing my own cannabis so I can be sure of how it is grown and the ratio of THC-CBD and also not waste my money, as it being illegal it is an expensive habit, one joint costs Â£3-5. Or if cannabis was sold legally at a reasonable price such as Â£10 an eighth or less

I would buy it. I think that vapourisers should be developed and be made affordable, at present they cost about Â£80. Vapourising is one of the best, healthiest, most efficient methods of using cannabis as only 4 percent of the THC is wasted as opposed to 76 percent in joints, there are no carcinogens, and actually cannabinoids have been proven to 'tell cancer cells to kill themselves.' I also use cannabis for period pain relief that is agonising, every position I am in the pain is unbearable. I cannot function with this pain, I can't even do simple tasks like coursework. The pain actually worries me because it feels like I may die, like a very dangerous pain. If I could describe this pain to you; I would say that it feels like my ovaries are going to explode, a little like extreme continual trapped wind, a very affecting sharp pain, it feels like I am bleeding to death. The pain is either completely vanished or very bearable depending on the variety after using cannabis. Cannabis is most effective in its herbal form. My favourite thing to do in life is climb a tree, sit at the very top, and spark dat zoobeeh!

287. Good questions.

288. Great stress reliever,very easy to grow and sell, most medicnal plant

289. great stuff, no harm at all.

290. Great survey

291. Habit forming but not addictive for me

292. had extream nerve pain from my cerical verbras Nothing I took from the doctors helped. But a friend said I should eat some

pot so we cooked it down in butter I took One teaspoon and 20mins later was finally in no pain that had been for 2years!! if had not found help I feel I wouldnt be here..

293. Has helped with with PTSD after being robbed at gun point by xxx men in my apartment, great for pain, helps me concentrate and get work done at both school and work.

294. Have smoked for 45 years. Two master's degrees, and a 37 yr career with AT&T. Smoked pot (almost) the whole time. Only rule was, never go to work high. Helps immensely with creativity in computer programming. After work, I would use pot, and come up with creative programming algorithms. Then I'd go the work the next day and write the code. My programs made Billions for xxxx (truly, estimates are 4-5 Billion!). After 45 years of smoking, I truly believe that MJ is the perfect miracle drug. Non addictive, can't kill you, no hangover, and great for your health. If everyone who drinks alcohol would have smoked pot instead, MILLIONS of lives would have been saved. MJ Works wonders for stomach problems and joint pain. First time I realized it was good for medical was when I had bad joint pain from taking Lipitor. Made it go away almost completely, but only while I was high (about 3-4 hrs). After that, pain returned. Works great for stomach cramps caused by bad food, gastroenteritis, etc. Makes pain and cramping go away in seconds. Does nothing for diarria from bad food though. My wife uses it for MS. Definitely helps her mental status. Also helps with muscle spasms. Wish we could get it legally in xxx. Going to CO in the summer so my wife can get medical advice from dispensaries , and we can maybe try different types based on that advice. Too bad we can't bring it back to xxx, but OK and KS are preying on people and stealing their money. What

right does the gov have to withhold medicine from my wife that could help her? She is miserable with the effects of MS. Thanks for your support in ending the drug war. People are suffering and dying. And the Drug War is destroying our young people's lives with criminal records.

295. Helps arthritis.

296. Helps me get thru the shitty parts of life

297. Helps me sleep. When I have had a busy day, it can be difficult to rest since I still have so much un needed activity in my head. Weed clears out these un needed thoughts, puts me in the moment, and helps me get the rest that I need.

298. Helps my stress and anxiety.

299. Helps pop my mind out of 'fuck I hurt' mode and into 'adventure' mode where I want to dance around, celebrating my existence, and make a difference in my life and the lives of others. Keeps my mind lubricated so I don't get stuck on any one thought to long. Helps me maintain my Zen. <3

300. Here were i live in Amsterdam, Netherlands things are not at all how it should be. It always was one of the leaders in the industry but gave their chances away. The medicinal values of cannabis are still not known to i would say at least 90% of the people. I'm starting a movement called xxxxxxxxxxxxxx in which i want to put cannabis in new light to let the people think and decide what it can mean for them or the people around them looking at the facts and research numbers. Dokters are getting involved and i hope to keep expanding the network and

movement internationally so we can eventually get this of the list of drugs with no medicinal values all over America but also in Europe it should be taken in new consideration.

301. How long do you typically wait before driving following Cannabis use? To answer this question better I should say I don't have a car so I never have to make a decision about this as public transit and my feet take me everywhere.

302. www.alchimiaweb.com/blogfr/cannabis-therapeutique/

303. http://www.encod.org/info/700-MEDICINAL-USES-OF-CANNABIS.html http://uknowledge.uky.edu/cgi/viewcontent.cgi?article=1026&context=pharmacy_etds www.karger.com/Article/FullText/356446#AC

304. I absolutely love and despise smoking dope. I feel I can't do anything without being stoned. I often feel paranoia and anxiety until I smoke and then I feel just like normal again. I wish I could give up everyday but obviously don't really want it enough to do it. It is addictive. It is a good pain relief so it should definitely be used for medical reasons. Although it makes people tired and unproductive, I have managed to sit through 4 years of Architectural Technology with smoking as much as possible everyday. I used it to reward myself for doing work and it worked. So it doesn't mean people can't do anything while smoking, if you can give yourself a kick up the arse you'll still get what you need done and you can still have your smokes in the evening. It is something I would like help in quiting but it's like a best friend at this stage and the thoughts of never smoking it again do scare me.

305. I actually live in California.

306. I also use as prescribed for migraine headache 3-4 times a year

307. I also use it to replace nsaids. Especially for cramps during menstrual cycle.

308. I also use it to treat headaches and had a prescription that expired but I primarily use it recreationally.

309. I am a hard working and faimly focased responsible individual. I am not a criminal even if the law says i am.

310. I am a 54-year-old educated, upper-middle-class white woman. I have been smoking marijuana since I was 15 years old. The only time I ceased smoking was during both of my pregnancies and six months thereafter, during breast-feeding. If I don't smoke marijuana, I am just a depressed, unmotivated person. I cannot seem to get going. Within five minutes of having one hit, I can focus and complete my daily tasks, which are many. As far as driving, it makes me more aware and focused. I do not speed when I smoke marijuana. When I go to sleep at night, I sleep uninterrupted for eight hours, at least. However, I do not smoke it before I go to my part-time job at a local elementary school because of the public stigma that it has. I do not understand why society readily accepts ingesting chemically -produced medicine in a lab with detrimental side effects, yet is so against a naturally grown plant that has many medicinal qualities and there is no processing whatsoever involved in the smoking of marijuana, and not nearly as many side effects.

311. I am a big proponent of medical cannabis. I have seen people

get CURED of cancer using it and I have seen people with MS get immediate relief. I have seen AIDS patient regain an appetite. I will sit back and watch for it to be recreational. I am not to sure about it being used by all people over 21. Don't get me wrong I don't think it will hurt them but they may not know how to dose and that could make people ill. I love growing my own Cannabis and I want to be able to continue to do that. Please don't close the Medical Cannabis places as I get good information from the staff.

312. I am a busy full time medical student and mostly use cannabis at night after my responsibilities are completed to relax. Sometimes I smoke when studying for boring topics which doesn't complicate my focus but makes it more bearable/ interesting. Cannabis can have either an increased or decreased effect on my motivation and energy depending on the social setting I am in, the time of day, and strain of cannabis. I often smoke at night which normally helps me sleep. However, sometimes it causes racing thoughts which make falling asleep more difficult. I have noticed that this habit of smoking at night does make early (6am) mornings more difficult.

313. I am a devoted cannabis activist and healer to the point of forgoing my own earnings as a CPA to engage in these activities. Well versed in the medical, historical, cultural and legal aspects of this fine botanical, I am often call into action through a growing network of cannabis activists to provide full treatments of full extract cannabis oil (concrete extract of cannabis) for critically ill children. My xxxxxxxxxx personna is well known for 'xxxxxxxxxxxxxxx Approximately 95% of xxxxxxxxxxx is donated free of charge and delivered throughout the nation to desperate parents. If you would like to know more about my

activities check xxxxxxxxxxxx on Facebook, or my company xxxxxxxxxxxxxxxxxxxxxxxx.

314. I am a doctor. I smoke a few joints twice a year. I allow time in between to limit impact on my memory. The criminalisation of marijuana is archaic. Any drug consumed to excess is damaging. If alcohol is legal and I can prescribe opiates, then surely we must make this drug legal. Legalisation is key to limiting negative impacts of the drug. People are using it irrespective of its legality, if it were legalised we could educate, control and tax it.

315. I am a full time graduate student living in Washington state.

316. I am a full time student and work a full time schedule. I enjoy marijuana responsibly, I turn to marijuana for a spirtual experience and because it improves my general well being.

317. I am a full-time student in a college town. I use cannabis both socially and privately. I have a hard time studying after I smoke so I enjoy it as a treat after studying! It helps me wind down but it is sometimes hard to sleep because I have a creative mind during its effects.

318. I am a graduate student in a medical school program. I don't find Cannabis hinders my ability to learn in anyway. It is useful to stay focused, eat regularly, and maintain stress and anxiety. Vaporizers are my preferred administration source but the devices are expensive so I smoke joints instead and notice I have a slight wheeze and low endurance in relation to joint smoking. I have smoked since I was 18 with only 1 year break. During these years I smoke anywhere from 3x week to 5x/day,

depending on my responsibilities. I find it easy to balance my responsibilities with my use. Cannabis makes me more clear mentally in heated discussions in my relationships, it keeps me calm and collected. I used Cannabis as a way to stop smoking cigarettes and chose it over other drugs like heroin, cocaine, or ecstasy during the few months I tried those drugs. I find hot baths sometimes increased the sedative effects of cannabis but also work together to calm me and reduce pain. I respect my herb by curing it in glass jars, I ALWAYS buy organic local product and will not buy anything but that. I do believe if I smoke too much, it reverses the effects to where I feel sober. Too little smoke makes me alert but jittery, my skin and nerves feel zingy! I prefer purple blends. I have grown it myself. I find an oral mucosal spray (orange dream) INSTANTLY helped me with severe seasonal allergies!!!! I also smoke with hemp twine vs. a butane lighter. I find no problem not smoking its just a bummer if I don't have flowers and I have nausea or am really stressed. It is SO helpful for regulating my period and menstrual cramps!

319. I am a high energy, anxiety driven person by nature. Cannabis slows me down, gives me patience and clarity, to carry out tasks and live a more enjoyable life.

320. I am a later in life user- I didn't try cannabis until I was 30. It has brought a lot of pain relief for chronic pain due to my endometriosis.

321. I am a long time cancer challenge. I wanted off of prescription pain meds. I didn't realized I was depended upon them until I went cold turkey and stopped them. The reason I was on them become magnified to the point I researched what I could

do to wean myself off the pharmaceutical world. I turned to Cannabis for the first time in my life. I am finally prescription meds free!

322. I am a medical patient, I have been sick for ten years and last year following a massive seizure, the right side of my body was paralyzed. I started Cannabinoid Therapy two months ago and I have more than 50 square inches of sensation in my effected side since starting treatment!

323. I am a mother of a 1 1/2 year old. My husband and I both smoke, but rarely at the same time unless we have someone to watch our son.

324. I am a paraplegic with sever neuropathic pain and spasms. I used prescription medications for 12 years with limited relief. I decided to try cannabis again (I had used it for about 10 years after college and then stopped for well over a decade) after reading about the medical benefits. My pain is greatly controlled as are my spasms. I have a much improved overall outlook on life. I began exercising regularly. After using it for the last 15 months I feel better than I have in the past 12 years, both physically and mentally. I am in the best physical shape since my paralysis. It has changed my life for the better significantly. My prescription drug use has greatly decreased. The positive change in my quality of life is greatly noticeable by friends and family. If only I would have discovered that it would help me a long time ago I wouldn't have had to suffer so much.

325. I am a physician who uses medical marihuana for multiple sclerosis symptoms in a state where it is not legal. I am often

afraid of random drug tests at work and frustrated when I cannot openly recommend what I May thing is the best treatment for my patient.

326. I am a social drinker who rarely gets 'drunk'. I stop at three drinks. I prefer cannabis over any other recreational mood enhancer and rather than any pain medication or sleep aid on the market. All I have to do is look at the pages of caveats and warnings telling me what will happen if I take the pharma drug. I believe that cannabis was made illegal to make it easier for the authorities to arrest people of color and to promote alcohol sales. Making it legal was the first smart thing about fighting the cartels this country has ever done.

327. I am a stage 4 peritoneal cancer patient and find cannabis is sometimes the only thing that helps the pain related to a year of chemo. I had used cannabis in college with little use between then and now (62 YOA). I probably would not use if I wasn't sick.

328. I am a stay at home mom. I used MM everyday during both of my pregnancies and while breastfeeding. The amout that I smoke depends on the quality...if its commercial/regs I use about 3/4 oz...if its medical grade about 1/4 oz. If I don't use MM my heart defect makes my life intolerable, I can't function like a normal person and member of society. MM improves my life incredibly.

329. I am a TBI (Traumatic Brain Injury)survivor, have used cannabis since 2001 for my injury. It has been the most effective medicine I have become aware of for treating my seizures, with range from tremors to full gran mals, cannabis has been

working so well, that I have completed over 10,000 miles of bicycling, which i was told I was not medically fit to undertake :)

330. I am a vocal opponent of prohibition.

331. I am a young cannabis smoker from California. I am very aware of the positive effects the usage of cannabis has and I think a lot of Californians do. However, as stoners are increasing and the use of marijuana is slowly but surely becoming more acceptable in modern society, I believe it's also VERY important that the proper information is out there. People need to realize that cannabis isn't for everyone and there are very well negative effects that could and have the potential to affect our lives as we know it. Cannabis activists always try to justify it with, 'it's just a earth made plant' and what have you but people need to know that there are repercussions to ANY type of indulgence and in excess. There's still a skill set of self control needed to handle marijuana despite people's belief of it 'not' being addictive. (I think cannabis is more 'dependent' than 'addictive,' however those are just technicalities) Those are my two cents, hope everything goes well with this survey.

332. I am alive today because of cannabis. I believe it will be a good change for our future to decriminalize.

333. I am all for legal recreational use. Colorado is on the right track with their program and it seems to be working out in their favor. Give the government a way to earn some tax dollars and me a way to enjoy my weekends.

334. I am all for legalization of cannabis on recreational and medical

levels as I have struggled with depression and anxiety issues since I was about 10 years old and it is the only thing that has actually helped that I didn't abuse to an extent it hurt my lively hood. It's a great thing, and should no longer be discriminated against for accusations brought on years ago by uninformed, scared people.

335. I am allergic to alcohol. Cannabis works better as a social drug and for a few conditions that I would rather not use drugs like Valium that I have been prescribed for. It eases anxiety and some symptoms of hypomania that I have so that I slow down and can take a step back from the pace I have worked myself up to. I have a very successful life and it has helped me a lot.

336. I am an MD. Despite it being illegal, I am very aware of the usefulness of cannabis. It helps my migraines and overall level of stress tremendously.

337. I am bipolar II and nothing improves my mood, outlook, quality of life, and cognitive function quite like cannabis does. I have been a doctor recommended medical marijuana patient for nearly 4 years, and in that time I have lost 55 lbs, replaced prozac and lorazepam, and have escaped the threat of high bp and cholesterol meds.

338. I am completely against 'labeling' the uses of, and the commodification of cannabis. I wish there were more information available for this survey to understand more specifically what outcomes you're looking for. Your survey questions regarding short term effects are inadequate / flawed simply because most cannabis users have medicated with both indica & sativa strains and everyone knows that these induce

vastly differing effects on the user. What information do you derive from me answering that my motivation is both increased & decreased when I medicate? This survey was befuddling.

339. I am conflicted on the question on whether it is addictive or not. I can quit if I have to but I don't want to. Its because I don't want to quit that I find it difficult. Example: I need a new job, in order to get one I have had to quit. But I am not enjoying being without it.

340. I am convinced this plant can save the Country.

341. I am currently an undergraduate student at the University of xxxxxxxxxxx double majoring in Economics and Finance. I began using cannabis one year ago. I have no medical need for cannabis, but school can get stressful and it is a nice release. Although I smoke 3 to 4 times a week, it has never taken over my life or negatively impacted my life. Overall my health has improved since I have started smoking in comparison to before I smoked. I assume this is mostly because of my decrease in consumption of alcohol. Although I understand that cannabis can certainly have negative impacts on peoples' lives, mine is not one of them

342. I am currently stopping smoking. I am into health and do extended periods of fasting and fruit diet, and have noticed that weed smoking is harmful to my body in these states as I evolve in my health pursuits. Also, I have an addiction to smoking weed in that I love to spend time smoking and it wastes money, leads to health effects, and take away from my personal and career endevours. At times in my life smoking cannabis has given me motivation and inspiration, the drive

to meditate and get into yoga, and encourage me intellectually and artistically. Therefore, I feel it is a healthier alternative to many other things, and it serves its purpose which for some may mean a lifetime and for others just for a period of time. I do have difficulty quitting, and money has been a major factor in increasing my interest to quit. I feel that it is a safer alternative then many other things and should be completely decriminalized, although that does not make it a 'healthy' thing to do.

343. I am currently taking paxil, buspar, and propranolol for anxiety. I did not put the effects of cannabis because it depends upon the strain - I get serious anxiety and panic attacks from high thc, so I no longer use that kind. Also, I used to be a daily smoker, but then I quit for several years and only recently started using it again for medicinal reasons.

344. I am ex-military and a veteran of the Iraq war, I have a great job with good benefits now. It's been quite a wild ride getting to where I'm at today. I was motivated by friends and my wife. I believe Cannabis helped me by cutting through all the BS and showing me myself for who I really am, not all the egotistical things that I believed and built to create some image that i though needed to show to the world. It helps me understand that behind all the ego we have created in this world, that we are really all the same; spiritual beings. Cannabis, as well as many other focuses like yoga, healthy eating, self acceptance and letting go of fear has been my biggest help dealing with trauma of war and a contradicting world of fear and drama.\ Hope this helps.

345. I am far more of a aggressive out of control driver without

Cannabis. In fact the only accident I have been in was when I did not have thc in my system.

346. I am glad you are doing this!

347. I am grateful for Ricks oil and keeping medical marijuana dedicated separate from recreational (I still substitute teach sometimes and public opinion doesn't 'get' this great medicine and judge those that use)It is important that it is tested for microbial and values of CBD and THC. I can not risk low blood pressure with high THC and do not like the effects of feeling high, altered too much and ineffective. It is important to understand the actual medicinal effects inside our bodies parameters. I also had a CDC counseling degree and use to to put kids in treatment. I do not like the youth using it for these reasons: addiction, use to avoid dealing with healthy problem solving skills, not developed brain, often driving and or practicing unsafe sex and lowered reasoning skills. It can be a false sense of social skills or self medication that needs better strategies. I have friends using it for pain mug, or cancer treatment nausea and are also needing to use AND be separated places for buying as they are very public figures.

348. I am happy with my cannabis use.

349. I am in favor of the legalization of Cannabis. I believe it can replace prescription drugs and treat many disorders, diseases, and even all forms of cancer. So many can benefit from this wonderful plant! :) Rock on, guys!

350. I am kinda different case as I was in the military for a decade and recently got out. I smoked a lot as a teenager but stopped

when I was 19. I have been experimenting with it since my departure from the military. I am one of those people that likes to catch a buzz on a friday night after a long work week. I prefer cannabis to alcohol, however, due to it's legal status in my state I do not plan on continued use. If it was legal, I would do it every weekend and occasional evening.

351. I am NOT a recreational user. I have advanced prostate cancer and am using a concentrated, alcohol solvent extracted thc/cbd Oil. I have relcated to Washington (along w/ my wife) so that I can have LEGAL access to Cannabis medicine. I have pursued this route of treatment at my oncologist's suggestion (xxxxx University hospital, xxxxxxxxx.), after both surgery and radiation failed to cure my cancer.

352. I am one of many people who consider this plant a miracle. I would not have survived this long if I were still dependent on legal drugs that dulled my personality & intelligence. Cannabis doesn't impair me, it reduces my pain to the level that I can function as if I didn't have the pain in the first place. I will be moving to Colorado within a year so that I don't have to be considered a criminal for taking my medicine.

353. I am peri menopausal and cannabis use decreases my symptoms.

354. I am prescribed an incredibly high amount of Vyvanse and Adderall. I don't know if this affects my 'high' when i smoke but it seems to make me more capable of utilizing the creativity that stems from my ADD while still maintaining the social and mental awareness that my medication helps me with. I smoke recreationally - only when the opportunity is presented - but unlike many of my peers, I do not like to get much more than

a light buzz. Regarding addiction, many of my friends that are under 18 (and have a green card) have struggled with excessive use of weed. They claim that they are not addicted but the availability of weed makes it hard for them to say no to the opportunity to get high. Conversly, most of these individuals struggle with depression or anxiety and simply view Cannabis as their medication and feel that being high most of the day is good for their mental health.

355. I am self medacaited i have been for many years but some times its hard to find with cops busting in the door of cannabis seller and not the meth heads... But i hope this helps with research . I use it for adha, pain, and annxitey i also get mingrines. But the street quality is nothing like the medical stuff.

356. I am so thankful for cannabis. Without side affects I can manage my pain and live life again! No more damage from prescription morphine!

357. I am temporarily disabled. I had surgery on my knee from a skiing accident thus am temporarily out of work. I also am in the process of moving back to Washington, I was previously living in Colorado. So I plan to be part time and eventually full time employed following the healing of my injury (as I was prior to surgery)

358. I am unclear if marijuana is addictive or not because I have used it almost daily for 10 years, before being an adult. I can say it's much easier to stop smoking marijuana than it is to quit smoking cigarettes, which I have done. I believe that any act or behavior can become addictive, not just substances. So, I'm still exploring this as I await more results from scientific studies

like this one. I believe that paranoia and decreased social skills arise not from the substance itself, but from the fear of social consequences. As it becomes legal, it will be interesting to see how anxiety levels are effected. Thank you for your dedication to this very important subject!

359. I am unemployed for the first time since i was 15. Although my schooling is limited, that does not mean to say i have not educated myself. I go through periods of smoking a lot and then periods of smoking nothing. I prefer marijuana to any anti-depressant/anxiety medication. I have been recommended medications in the past and refused and with the use of my mind and positive steps within myself (also using cannabis when i've felt it would help and have had the funds) through this i believe i have battled a lot (more than the milder reasons people are prescribed opiates) caused by the use of other drugs by my parents. I do not use any drug other than alcohol or marijuana, i have in the past but do not feel the need any more. I believe marijuana is addictive if abused but i see more of a mental tie than physical and i think that with education and naturalisation people can use it to heal rather than abuse.

360. I am very allergic to pain meds, muscle relaxers and many RX products, I use cannabis instead with better relief and no side effects.

361. I am very sensitive to strain & THC content, so have to select carefully. Some types are deeply relaxing, while others may cause extreme oversensitivity and/or intense, full-body, nerve pain.

362. I am willing to discuss this with you in person if I can be of

any help with your endeverours regarding Medical Marijuana. I am in range of and know where your school is located. I will check with the office to see if your protocol allows you to speak with participants. So, very happy you are doing this study. Please, Israely Doctors have done years worth of clinical trails. So have the British.

363. I answered a few of the questions about the effects with conflicting answers because the effects vary quite a lot depending on the situation and what activities I am engaged in. More of a situation amplifier than distorter.

364. I answered cannabis is motivating and is demotivating. While immediate effect is motivating, after effect wears off, which is usually fairly quickly for me this becomes a relaxing unmotivated period where I can easily go right to bed without tossing and turning or at the very least sit and watch a movie with my wife or get some reading in. I think it's hard sometimes to separate self prescribed medicinal use and recreational use as I also use regularly as a preventative for many chronic conditions for which it has been shown to help.

365. I attribute cannabis to my increased quality of living.

366. i be live through patterned use cannabis relives my back pain and helps me get fullnight sleep

367. I been a mmj patient since 2000. my civilian dr prescribed it to me. I started making thc hash oil (phoenix tears) It has kept me cancer free for 14 years. Also no man-made narcotic pills since 2000 either. I no longer have muscle spasms, pain in my back and arthritis pain in all my joints and muscles. Love not

having the side effects and drugged out feeling the next day on prescription pills.

368. I began using cannabis for anxiety & insomnia relief. But its benefits have gone beyond my expectations. For me it is definitely a healing plant. Often while using cannabis I become very happy, content, and relaxed, but sometimes I get highly emotional, introspective, and need to be alone and think. I've realized, after 3 years of use, that Cannabis is able to help me become more aware of certain trauma in my past and how it has affected me as a developing person. I feel more comfortable and capable in confronting these difficult memories/ personal issues. I have successfully been able to release old hurtful patterns of thinking/ behavior. It aids me in counseling/therapy to really deal with challenges in my mental & emotional health and practice how to overcome challenges. I believe cannabis gives me a bigger perspective and deeper understanding of myself. This perspective in turn frees me to understand and connect better with others.

369. I began using cannabis recreationally from the age of 18 at 27 I had a bad motorcycle accident which left me with nerve damage to my right leg and since then I have used cannabis to control the pain and muscle spasms.

370. I began using cannabis recreationaly when I was 15. However, when I was 24 some nerve endings in my back broke and cannabis has been the only pain medication that has been not only effective but that does not have such negative side effects. Before I switched to medical cannabis, the prescription pain medicine I tried made me too sick and tired to function normally. The side effects of cannabis, however, are actually

positive (people recreationaly use cannabis for the effects that I consider to be side-effects because my primary motivation for use is pain management, but the side-effects are still the positive ones associated with a marijuana high. Cannabis has been the only pain drug that I have found that doesn't have a tolerance issue (I've used the same two or three hits per time as an effective dose for almost a year, whereas for Vicodin I had to increase my dosage fairly early on and several times before I finally gave up on it) and cannabis is simply more effective as a pain management drug for the sort of long term chronic nerve pain that I suffer from. I think cannabis certainly has recreational value, but its primary use and understanding should be medical. Also, not every strain is effective for pain management. In fact, most strains, especially sativa dominate strains, do very little for pain. Pure CBD cannabis doesn't work very well either, there needs to be a combination of THC and CBD for maximum pain relief. Other than that, I use cannabis several times a day and have for years. While I would not recommend such heavy use for students or others that need to study books and remember everything, I have had no problems with heavy use effecting my work and I work as a campus security officer. Actually, part of the reason I switched to cannabis for pain management is that I realized that I am more alert, functional, and on top of my game (which is necessary for medical and criminal response) with cannabis in my system than any other prescription drug the doctors gave me.

371. I began using High CBD cannabis to eventually replace the pain medication (Dilaudid) that is in my intrathecal implanted pain pump. I am only three weeks away from putting saline into my pump, thus not using Dilaudid at all. I could not be doing this without CBD cannabis. I am still limited to only

certain activities with my upper body, but I am not in the intense, tortuous pain I was in before starting CBD therapy. My naturopathic doctor prescribed what to use. I only use the capsules, vaporizer, and topicals at this point. My pain level is down 50% plus. Time will tell after I have the Dilaudid taken out of my pump - how much cannabis I will need. This is a miracle to me after 15 years of disability and chronic use of prescription medications.

372. I believe alcohol is much more dangerous than cannabis and ruins many more lives.

373. I believe Cannabis can be addicting to some, but not all people. That wasn't clear in the answer sections.

374. I believe cannabis has many medical benefits. I also believe that a lot of the people with medical cards use it for recreation purposes, which doesn't bother me because I am pro legalization. Although I do not believe that Cannabis is physically addictive I do believe for some people it can be psychologically addictive.

375. I believe cannabis has more positive qualities than negative ones and should be legalized.

376. I believe cannabis has numerous medical usages. For me, personally, it improves my sleep quality drastically. Without cannabis, I awaken at least six times per night and have difficulty falling back asleep. With cannabis, this number is one or zero. If I do awaken, I use cannabis to immediately fall back asleep. In these circumstances, I use a heavy indicated, high CBD strain. I also use cannabis to alleviate acute anxiety, depression and aid in concentration. For these purposes, I use a high thc

70-90% sativa. The strains which a primarily use are Critical Mass (high CBD) and Bubba Kush(heavy indica) for sleep and pain, Sour Diesel or purple diesel for anxiety and depression and Golden Goat for focus and concentration. It is critical that I choose the correct strain, as they all have completely different effects.

377. I believe cannabis is a great medical product along with recreational use, I have used both alcohol and cannabis and I have experienced a better quality of life on cannabis, it I motives my depression greatly and allows me to eat a healthy diet

378. I believe cannabis is a safer choice for medication for my pain and depression. It works as well as the prescriptions (or better) and is not addictive or dangerous to the other systems in my body. I am sad that it is illegal in my state and wish I could move to where it is legal, but currently I cannot.

379. I believe cannabis is a true gift for the world and its use should be widespread and frequent. We need to study the endocannibinoid system more to understand disease.

380. I believe cannabis is a useful tool that can impart many benefits. It is safer than alcohol. The hemp plant has many uses, as a fiber for clothing, for building material, as nutritional product, as in hemp milk. I am sad that the promoters of the legalization initiative were so shortsighted and dishonest about the measure. MMJ and industrial hemp are valuable products.

381. I believe cannabis isn't for everyone, it will be negative for some and positive for others, what is important is our choice, our sovereign right to choose how we perceive the world and what

state of consciousness we live in. There is a lot of misinformation about cannabis and should be approached with an open mind, like all things in life.

382. I believe cannabis to be psychologically addictive, as opposed to physically addictinve. It CAN make you boring, and take away motivation if you use it as an escape to your problems (just like any other drug, including alcohol, icecream, chocolate....) It makes you content with being boring because it allows you to be entertained by just about anything. It amplifies your emotions. If you're happy you'll feel extatic. If you feel sad, it might make it worse if you create a negative environment with depressing music.

383. i believe cannabis to be the most beneficial thing on the face of this earth and was put here to cure or treat almost any ailment that prescription drugs(pills) 'say' they cure while only causing further damage to the human body. also thank you fr making this survey i hope it helps open peoples eyes to how good it can be and maybe oneday be legal worldwde so everybody can share true happiness PEACE LOVE and LEGALIZE have a good day whom ever is reading this! TOKE IT UP!

384. I believe in cannabis as an incredible medicine. There is no medicine more effective or SAFER than cannabis. I also believe in the use of cannabis during pregnancy as opposed to any anti - nausea or pain medicines.

385. I believe in cannabis as medicine. I do not live in an mmj state, so all I can get is what I can get on the black market. I would LOVE to be able to chose my strain and use concentrates to appropriately medicate. As it stands, I get a strain and I try

it. If the initial anxiety is too high to outweigh the medicinal factor, I cannot use it. My husband is both recreational and medicinal, and he likes all kinds, as long as it is potent. It used to be, we could only get Mexican pressed weed. Now, we know a grower. But it is very very small so there is no strain variation. I do like that we are no longer supporting a dangerous source/ structure and now are just helping our friends. But We need mmj in Ohio. I believe in recreational legalization also, but I believe that medical must be in place to give patients some level of protection. Also cannabis MUST be rescheduled!! It is INHUMANE to deny nontoxic medicine to people and push poison onto them as their only legal possibility for relief!!

386. I believe in Cannabis, and you should too. It's truly a wonderful plant.

387. I believe it has helped me with anxiety, bodily aches and pains, relaxes my mind and encourages peacefulness.

388. I believe it is therapeutic and awesome recreationally or as a hobby. The medicinal and social pros outweigh the cons.

389. I believe people should have the right to consume cannabis for enjoyment and as medicine.

390. I believe smoling cannabis helps to relax you after all the angst of the day. I tjink cannabis is lless harmful to society than alcohol.

391. I believe that 'addictive' traits can be found in ANY/ALL substance/s. You can become addicted to McDonalds!! I have been and stopped eating it and felt sick for a week!!! I believe

that most addictions are psychological and it stems from a need to feel a part of something or to cover an emotional imbalance in their life. I DO NOT believe that cannabis is 'addictive' but I DO believe you can become addicted! People become dependent of everything including other people. Cannabis is a very beneficial PLANT and it has such a wide range of medicinal purposes as well as spiritual applications. I believe that this 'drug war' is a total failure. Cannabis has helped me a lot with connecting to my spiritual path and lift my consciousness level over the years. It has also been beneficial in dealing with the emotional chaos that has engulfed the American people with poverty and ignorance and any and all parts of their government. Truth is I have found more cannabis users in states where it is Illegal than in the states where it is legal. I live in Colorado and the average age for a 'red card' holder or a medicinal cannabis patient is 42! Simply put Cannabis should be taken off Schedule 1 for the following reasons. A. It does have Medicinal benefits! B. It does have emotional/psychological benefits. C. It is not Addictive or habit forming. D. We can create a surplus in our government $$$$-1. not jailing people for petty cannabis charges. 2. By taxing the current systems and users implemented on a State level. E. Create a safer America by suffocating the illegal market forcing them out of the U.S. or forcing them to become a legitimate entity thus creating even more work and taxes to circulate into our economy!! Thanks. Soon we will all be free of the metaphorical chains of Oppression and be able to live in a country of true and undeniable FREEDOM! I have faith in our country to find true peace as well as to become a well informed society of free thinkers!!

392. I believe that cannabis is a wonderful option for so many different conditions and is something I am very passionate

about. Cannabis should be legal on a federal level and I think it should be utilized by so many that are suffering. I believe it is a much better choice than a lot of toxic pharmaceuticals prescribed.

393. I believe that cannabis itself is a non-addictive substance, but that people may become addicted to the feelings associated with ingesting it. If I feel I'm consuming more than I should, I have no problem stopping for a while.

394. I believe that it should be the sovereign right of every adult to choose to smoke cannabis if they wish to do so. The war on drugs is a war of greed and monopoly.

395. I believe that marijuana's propensity for causing anxiety/ paranoia is linked to it's legal status. Since getting my prescription, I feel these effects less often, but they Seem to be happening with less frequency.

396. I believe that oral administration of fixed-oil extractions like 'cannabutter' requires more research for safe dosing.

397. I believe that recreational use of cannabis is a good thing and it will help our economy if we make it legal across our country.

398. I believe the 'addictive' nature of cannabis is primarily habitual/ psychological rather than based in a physiological dependence.

399. I believe there should be more research and study to see where cannabis can be used in the place of other heavily prescribed medications.

400. I believe this plant keeps me sane and happy. It should be made available to everyone without restrictions. Name just one drug that is safer..........

401. i broke my femur a few months ago - pain and mood, use of substances affected by this very much. full time student

402. i broke my neck last year and am eternally greatful for cannabis and its wonderful effects weening me off the hard pain meds.

403. I broke nine bones in my spine and would suffer a great deal without Cannabis, I wish not to be hidden in your test, my name is xxxxxxxxxxxxxxxxxxxxxxxxx and please use me in your test as much as you can. I want to help you folks better understand Cannabis and it's effects.

404. I can attest to the efficacy of MedCann for my patients (when working with Indian Health Service), and clients (everyone else). I have about 12 Vet friends (from Vietnam to Afghanistan/Iraq) who feel and use MedCann as an adjunct to their PTSD Tx. This whole plant medicine needs to be available to everyone. The decreased intrusive thoughts/nightmares, affect dysregulation, and numbing/avoidance/dissociation is reported to me and while I worn about overuse, I definitely see a difference between the Rx psychopharms use and MedCann use. Keep up the good work. I was at the xxxx Cannabis Therapeutics Conference in xx and was very impressed with the presenters and clinical studies. And I got to meet Dr. Michoulam! And do not get me started comparing MedCann to Rxs or ETOH and tobacco...sigh.

405. I can't fathom how marijuana is still illegal while cigarettes and

liquor (which are responsible for far more deaths) are legal.

406. I clicked a bunch of contradictory short term effects, because different strains do contradictory things depending on which you're smoking. Also, as for the symptoms of cannabis 'withdrawal,' I'm pretty sure in almost every instance it's just people annoyed they don't have any more weed. Like if you can't sleep without weed, it's not a withdrawal, it just means you've let yourself get used to sleeping high and now you need to adjust. Same with me being irritable, it's pretty much just boredom caused by not being able to get high. I don't like the term 'withdrawal' when referring to weed at all, and I think if you did a study on TV 'addicts' you'd find they have nearabouts the same symptoms as cannabis 'addicts' when going through 'withdrawals.'

407. I credit the use of cannabis to a vast improvement in my mental health and self esteem during my teenage years.

408. I currently work a camp job, so while I do partake heavily on my days out of camp I am completely sober two weeks out of the month while I'm in camp, I usually don't feel any withdrawal symptoms but when I do get home my tolerance has completely dropped.

409. I decided to quit smoking....again... on August 30th. I've been using pot on and off since I was 16 y/o...43 years. I'm having a very hard time dealing with my life now. I smoked to feel better, to deal with my anxiety and depression and feel connected in a spiritual way. I substituted getting high for developing another spiritual practice like meditation or yoga, though I've practiced both on and off all my life. For years I

smoked before work as well as when I got home. Pot has been my companion for most of adult life. I've used to deal with abdominal and gynecological pain, as well as mental health issues. I quit because I was feeling worse, more anxiety, very confused and choking. I'm working with a psychologist and taking 5HTP and Omega 3's to help find balance in my life. I'm sending this in and will write to the researchers to see if there's more specific help for me. I have loved pot and now I look back and see I used it to escape my responsibilities. I failed to plan financially and am living in financial crisis. I am an addictive personality. For others who can moderate their use, it appears to be a very good thing. At this point I feel I've been impacted negatively by my lifelong use as my physical and mental health are poor. Thanks for doing this survey and giving me space to comment.

410. I did indicate that I work full time (two jobs). I did before moving to enter a full time graduate school program.

411. I did not touch marijuana after quittting in college until both my life became unbearable AND Seattle had dispensaries. I did not want to have a 'drug dealer' and do not consider myself a drug abuser.

412. I didn't smoke cannabis for years, because it just made me an introvert. But as I've entered my forties and started having some sleep issues, and other hormonal issues, I have found it very useful for getting to sleep and relieving migraines.

413. I didn't start using every day until I moved to Seattle. I was really depressed and had no friends. I was a student so I had a lot of down time. I have found that it helps me to focus while

studying. It may take me longer but I can focus for longer periods of time while high.

414. i discovered marijuana rather late, at the age of 30. i have mild asthma so i can't smoke. i have a prescription for marijuana and the edibles have worked wonders for me. they make me more relaxed and put me in a better, creative mood. also, as i age, i find that i need less to equal the same effect, so for me, it's the opposite of addictive. i'm so glad and thankful that prohibition is ending. don't forget: our US constitution is printed on hemp paper and george washington grew it!

415. i do have a prescription for it and i'm delighted that the prohibition against it has ended in my state (wa).

416. I do not believe that cannabis itself is addictive, it is habit forming just almost anything is to human beings. Someone that becomes a heavy regular smoker of cannabis is likely to have had some reason to be doing it, and if it wasn't cannabis it would have been something else

417. I do not consider marijuana addicting because when I need to, I am able to stop smoking marijuana without any withdrawl/ negative symptoms at all

418. I do not drive so those questions pertaining to driving were n/a Also, I choose my cannabis based mainly upon availability, which was not listed in the question on selection criteria

419. I do not frequent mmj dispensaries, prefering my friends or my own small, private - presently affirmatively defensible under 69.51a - gardens.

420. I do not think it is addictive although many people I know well who have smoked for 4 years or more everyday must smoke in order to feel hungry to eat and must smoke to feel happier. I think it affects dopamine levels over years of usage. Indica calms me and Sativa make me stay up and worry. I have had spiritual hallucinations many times I felt I was dying in which the most severe from taking a knife hit of hash and other times from edibles. I now have been able to control the hallucinations by drinking water and eating throughout the high. Smoking absolutely makes music sound better, food taste better and helps me relax during sex. During menstruation hash oil is the only substance that takes the pain of cramps away. Smoking helps to focus better watching movies but worse while reading.

421. I do not think that by itself that cannabis would be able to do more than dull pain and such. I do, however, fully belieeve that combined with other medications it can help to boost preventative and cures.

422. I do not think that if you just have recreational goals for cannabis is addictive, but medical use it is for the sole reason of: 'I would not stop vaporizing cannabis because I do not want my pain to come back.' Wanted to put a note on that.

423. I do not think the substances in marijuana are addictive. I think the sense of peace and euphoria sought by the user is addictive and found in the use of thc. I don't understand why it helps me focus, motivate and fight depression. I have opposite effects from many of my peers.

424. I do not use cannabis to get high, I use it to control various pains. some of them it controls better than others I mainly

use tinctures and and topical ointments. I did not answer the questions n smoking it because I have not smoked cannabis since 1987.

425. I don't believe cannabis is addictive in a chemical way. I think if someone is predisposed to being addicted, they may abuse cannabis the same as one might overindulge in food, exercise or alcohol.

426. I don't believe Cannabis is addictive, I believe it is habit forming. I've been smoking on and off for about 7 years now and it's never caused a decline in health or mental faculty, while helping me manage physical and mental trauma. If abused I think it can probably cause some problems, but each person is different and it affects everyone differently.

427. I don't believe Cannabis itself is addictive. People with addictive tendencies can have problems with it, just as people get addicted to coffee. It's just an altered state that they enjoy. The Chemicals aren't forcing their brains to crave it for seemingly no reason like tobacco or hard drugs. The fact is that it may be addictive to some, but it is not chemically addictive.

428. I don't believe in the idea of 'recreational' use. Most folks will tell you that they use cannabis because it makes them feel better. Feeling better shouldn't be thought of as recreational. I consider it a wellness tonic.

429. I don't believe Marijuana is a gateway drug. Some people begin using harder drugs to escape something and most follow because friends are using harder drugs. I went to rehab for pain killers and weed has no trigger for me to relapse.

430. I don't believe my Cannabis use is 'recreational', which implies using it for fun. I enjoy Cannabis because of the way it changes my perceptions and heightens my senses. In this regard, I think the term 'spiritual' may be more relevant.

431. I don't drive much currently as I live in New York City but in the time I have spent living elsewhere I have never experienced a problem with cannabis impairing my driving. It is most effective for me as a remedy for the occassional bouts of depression I experience as a result of adolescent traumas. I adore it for its creative function but I try to avoid everyday use in order to retain my ability to dream vividly. Also I have recently begun using sugar kief tincture and tend to prefer that to smoking, particularly because I am around three months clean from tobacco.

432. I don't know much about it but am looking into it more for migraine and stress relief.

433. I don't like the feeling of being high. I don't like my mind bein altered. I live in a state where medical cCannabis is legal.

434. I don't live in Washington State and I wish I did live in a state that had medical marijuana use. Working on that fight and we'll be there eventually.

435. I don't smoke to 'feel cool' or to 'escape', I smoke to help improve my quality of life. without it, I am a miserable, negative person who gets too deep into my own mind fR too often. marijuana helps me see that life isn't as bad as I think it is. With it I am able to sleep through the night, I've started school and work full time, and I'm engaged to be married all thanks in part to the

motivation it gave me to stop dwelling on the past and move on and so something with the life I was given.

436. I don't think cannabis itself is addictive. There have been times where it was ridiculously easy for me to lay off. I think that we are creatures prone to making things easier on ourselves and have a great potential for relying on such things, (some more than others) and it just so happens that cannabis does a good job at that, but is by no means the one to blame. I also think that by labeling cannabis as recreational, it smudges the concept of medical by pairing it with substances such as tobacco and alcohol, (both substances with no medicinal value) and will change the way we view and use it. Many people of all professions and backgrounds were starting to come out of the closet and open their minds to a previously demonized herb because of the medical benefits and good intentioned-usage. Now that it is labeled as recreational and has been stuffed in the room with alcohol and tobacco - just another thing to get high on - I think we will begin see a much darker side of cannabis arise and slowly what was once a very promising medicinal plant for many ailments and many people will become swept under the rug as a substance that supposedly serves other purpose than to escape from reality. The way we use our words and language has a great effect on the way we perceive things. Bring back the sanctity of Medical Cannabis.

437. I don't think that cannabis is physically addictive at all, I think any dependency on it is mental and can be overcome if the person is in the right mindset. I also do not believe it is a gateway drug, I just think that people who are interested in experiencing the types of feelings you get on other drugs are just more comfortable with trying something natural like

cannabis first. just like anything else, excess is bad. Moderate use of cannabis is not detrimental to anyone's well being or quality of life.

438. I don't use it but everyone I know does. I think it should be legal for them as they use it for self medicating chronic pain.

439. I dont think there is anything wrong with recreational or medical use!!!\

440. I enjoy Cannabidiol and dabbing it. Use to use THC in extract form for ADD/ADHD but grown out of it.

441. I enjoy smoking cannabis

442. I enjoy the way cannabis makes me feel but I wouldn't smoke it if I thought it was harmful to my health. I feel better and sleep better when I do smoke or eat cannabis prior to going to sleep.

443. I enjoy using cannabis and it feels a lot safer and more mellow than drinking. I don't take other drugs but I think it can easily be seen as a gateway drug. However, I strongly believe that this isn't a fault of cannabis, but rather a social fault. Where I live it's illegal to consume cannabis, so to access it you need to find a dealer. This is what I believe leads to other drugs - the accessibility of finding dealers.

444. I feel as though people make a far bigger deal of cannabis anditit's uses than is necessary.

445. I feel cannabis is a completely non-addictive and unharmful substance that has endless medical capabilities. Not a single

reported death ever. Which means that it's safer than water. This incredible herb should be actively cultivated by everyone in the world. I believe it's prohibition has a lot to do with the companies who make so much money of the products that cannabis would make obsolete. Which are many.

446. i feel like cannabis should be legalized In my state so that I can get rid of my depression when I smoke it makes me forget about all the depression and makes me feel relaxed and calm

447. I feel marijuana effects my motivation, and this troubles me, but I am much less motivated without it. My stress level increases when I do not have access to marijuana, but I believe this to be more of an emotional attachment than physical addiction. I used to drink heavily, but rarely do now, as I have replaced that part of my life with moderate marijuana use. I almost never take any pills of any kind, including aspirin as I find cannabis is as effective for pain and has much more pleasant side effects.

448. I feel more depressed in the days following cannabis use.

449. I feel strongly that medical marijuana should be separated from recreational marijuana in terms of sales administration, farming, and research. I believe MM patients should be able to grow their own medicine.

450. I feel that Cannabis saved my life. I had to take so many pain killers to deal with an issue in my spine that I could not engage with the world. I switched to Cannabis, particularly high CBD strains and CBD oral delivery methods, and the pain subsided to a point where I could interact.

451. I feel that different weed makes you feel different ways.

452. I feel that it makes me a better person, all around. I am more patient and umderstanding, not stressed out by things. If i could afford cannabis on a more regular basis (as i can only afford it every 3 months), I feel my life would run much much more smoothly.

453. I feel that marijuana has gotten the nick name of a gateway drug because of the strong misconceptions caused by propaganda. I used to think it was the worst thing you could ever do, then I tried it and realized it was NOTHING like what I was taught growing up. That caused me to question the validity of what I was told about all recreational drugs but quickly learned that I hated most if not all of them and stopped trying them. I do not even like the feeling of being drunk. However, smoking marijuana has improved, yes, improved my pregnancy, improved my anxiety, improved the level of nausea I have when experiencing one of my many migraines with aura. I am 24 weeks along in my pregnancy and I have gotten nothing but rave reviews on the level of development my baby has gone through. I think it has a lot to do with keeping my anxiety at a minimum even during the worst pregnancy symptoms.

454. I feel that marijuana is a safer more affective way to treat certain medical conditions, as well as a better recreational option for me personally.

455. I feel there are more benefits to marijuana than cons

456. I find cannabis Extremely useful for attitude adjustment in this culture we live in. Vaporizors are a more healthy delivery system.

With just a small intake I can be present to what matters, which is love for all existence. The pot we grew up with in college (1970's) is far better potency nowadays. I have had too much intake, usually through edibles. There have been a couple times where I was incapable of normal responsibilities. Once this was due to a blend of alcohol and pot. I find the stigma associated with medical weed very unhelpful as there is such a need for elders and veterans, who need alternatives to pharmaceuticals.

457. I find it addictive when I have some, but if I don't have it, I don't seem to have a problem not smoking it. I would use it everyday if I have it, but I do notice problems with recall the next day and maybe the next couple of days after using it the night before. I notice this goes away after a week or so of no use. I would like to know more about it's long-term use affects, it may reduce how often I use it.

458. I find it addictive, but quitting is not hard if I decide to, like taking tolerance breaks.

459. I find it odd that I continue to use and 'want' cannabis despite the fact that it makes me feel intellectually impaired to some extent. Perhaps I like the way it makes my body feel or the way I appreciate art and music under its influence.

460. I find it to be great for everyday use, it heels emotional pain as well as physical pain, anxiety, boredom, ect.

461. I find it very relaxing and it helps me sleep and talk to people in social settings. I used to feel some paranoia, but after using it regularly that went away and I'm only left with the good effects.

Also helps really well with minor aches and pains, headaches etc.

462. i find it very useful to fall asleep regardless of how much caffiene i comsume or any other factors that would otherwise affect my sleep pattern negatively

463. I find myself less interested in taking other drugs since using Cannabis, in the past I was using dexamphetamines and ecstacy as party drugs combined with alcohol (on an irregular basis). Since using cannabis my alcohol use has dropped significantly and I've not used anything else. I find that alcohol can have a very negative impact on my mood and cause me serious spells of depression, cannabis on the other hand always lifts my mood and is an excellet way to wind down in the evenings. While taking cannabis I've managed to get down to a very healthy weight and maintain it alot easier than i ever have in the past. I've been using cannabis for about 1 year.

464. I find that cannabis it self is not addictive but the high it gives is. I have used other drugs to chase the high when cannbis isnt available.

465. I find that the day after using cannabis, their can be a strong feeling of lethargy/depression, as well as a craving or addictive feeling. These subside after one day.

466. I find using marijuana means i dont have to take big pharma drugs for sleep, pain and anxiety.

467. I firmly believe in cannabis as a medicine and a safer alternative to alcohol

468. I first started to regularly medicate because of God-awful menstrual cycles. Smoking up was the only thing that stopped the cramping, the crushing depression and fatigue I would feel during my cycles. Queen Victoria used it in the same fashion, so if it's was good enough for old Vicki, it's good enough for me.

469. I first started use at age 32. I have been diagnosed Bipolar II. My Cannabis use began in an effort to replace prescription pharmaceuticals for anxiety, depression, and manic episodes. After 10 month of stable use, I consider low dose Cannabis use to be the most effective treatment that I have found for my condition.

470. I frequently use cannabis to offset the effects of 'coming down' from my prescribed Vyvanse

471. I gave some answers that look contradictory, e.g., more motivated for physical activity and also less motivated for physical activity, and more energized/more peaceful. What I meant by those choices was: the level of physical activity is usually decided before I smoke weed and is enhanced by the weed, and that I can become more alert and feel more energized while retaining calmness and peacefulness. Insomnia is the biggest medical reason for my use, and I do dearly love to get high for fun. Also, I try to avoid getting drunk too often, so smoking weed is a good alternative when I need to alter my consciousness. I would like to say that altering one's state of consciousness is necessary for a healthy mind, and that many different forms of alteration--whether drugs or exercise or religion--can cause similar meta-effects, if not similar immediate effects.

472. I go in and out of phases with Cannabis. I smoke heavily for a period of a few months and really enjoy the way it makes me feel. It stimulates my interest in classes, reading, and just life in genera and energizes and motivates me. After a few months of heavy use, though, getting 'stoned' transforms into a numbing and often anxiety-inducing experience. When this happens, I stop consuming Cannabis for a few months. When I start up again, the positive experience returns.

473. I grew up in a bad environment as a kid and hadn't ever dealt with anything and had just avoided problems by being stoned all the time and when I sobered up my problems reared their head. I always assumed my cannabis use started it but I now believe it masked an already developing problem. I've tried a few different meds and found them to be effective but soul destroying. I had low blood pressure already and would feint if I woke up too early after having taken them the night before and After a month I started to feel like I'd had a lobotomy. I couldn't think straight and felt a slowing of my thoughts. Cannabis has all of the benefits but none of the downsides for me.

474. I grow High quality cannabis for myself and other patients. I grow three strains that are each medical. I grow a high Hawaiian Snow for it's high THC, Harlequin for it's 2:1 ratio CBD:THC, and AC/DC for high CBD only. This allows me to make a variety of concentrates,infused edibles and non psychoactive topical. I teach new patients how to find witch of these solution's fits their needs. I call myself a 'Cannabis Coach'

475. I grow medicinal cannabis for myself and 10 patients. I grow 3 strains, 1 high THC, 1 THC +CBD, 1 high CBD only plant. We use the entire plant of the three strains for flowers, concentrates,

topical salves, and butter for edibles. We make strain specific and blends of our plants to provide a wider range of solutions for our patients. 502 will not allow me to continue to provide care for my patients. Please Help protect our right to help each other.

476. I had a bad back injury when I was younger and took pain killers on a regular basis. When I was 17 I discovered weed and never looked back.

477. I had a problem with Cannabis dependence for five years post trauma. Used ayahuasca to stop successfully and now I only smoke on breaks from school because it greatly impairs my cognitive function for about two weeks post use.

478. I had a stomach virus a few weeks ago and cannabis stopped my vomiting and nausea. I usually cannot participate in social settings because more often than not people smoke 'spliffs' which are a mixture of tobacco and cannabis. I wish this weren't the case. Tobacco makes me sick, I hate the smell, and think it is very bad for your health. I really wish this weren't so common.

479. I had cancer I need this

480. I had hyperemisis when I was pregnant with my son and cannabis was the only thing without side effects that allowed me to eat and drink. My friends were prescribed pharmaceuticals for their nausea and their children have very unfortunate birth defects due to the drugs their mothers' doctors gave them.

481. I had sleeping problems all the way through my child hood, nothing helped tried all avenues. As soon as I found cannabis

my sleep was excellent, my life improved..and I found I could lower my dosage of Mirtazapine which was prescribed to me for Insomnia but also for depression. Cannibas opened my mind to so many different ways or learning and I owe my life to it.

482. I hardly drink alcohol anymore and just use cannabis because the effects are a lot more enjoyable, and alcohol gives me bad heart palpitations. Also I had to put unemployed, but i am a student working towards my degree, not someone that sits on the couch all day smoking.

483. I have (almost) no appetite; as such, I self medicate with cannabis so that I can eat more and a greater variety of foods (makes me a more adventurous eater; I'm usually VERY picky). I should clarify that I don't think cannabis is physically addicting; I do believe that it can be mentally addicting. I suspect I have ADD; I tend to focus better on school work or research when I'm high, so I included that as part of the 'medicinal' usage. I may have slight insomnia (trouble getting to sleep). Cannabis helps greatly to calm me and make me tired. There are conflicting boxes checked in the 'short term effects' section; I am pulling from all of my experiences of cannabis use, and considering CBD/THC ratios, and how that has affected me in the short term. I also have checked 'hallucinations' under the aforementioned section. This only happened on three separate occasions; the first was about 2 months into smoking every day, and happened because I had swallowed smoke into my stomach. The next time was after the month long hiatus mentioned in one of the sections, after I had taken a hit of oil concentrate that may have weight about 0.2 grams or more. The

third was during a smoking party, after I had smoked about 0.5 grams of oil concentrate.

484. I have a high pressure, well paying career in the heart of Seattle. We own several properties that keep us busy on the weekends. I would much rather relax with cannabis than alcohol, recreationally. And medically, I find that is much more effective for managing short term stress/insomnia/nausea than the myriad of OTC/Rx now available. Very thankful it is finally legal in our great state. Thank you, Washington.

485. I have a LOT of medical issues that I use marijuana for. I have horrific SI Joint Dysfunction and cannot move without cortisone injections and medicinal marijuana. I also am highly anxious and stressed, and all the prescribed meds in the world do not help the way marijuana does. I also have complicated GI problems, and often the only way to eliminate nausea and be able to eat is with marijuana. And finally, I have a genetic cancer disorder (Lynch Syndrome) for which I recently had a complete hysterectomy. I do not have cancer at this point but could at any time in any number of locations. I fully believe in the powers of marijuana to help fight cancer so that is a factor in my use. I do not use any marijuana before having to do anything outside the home, never driving or at work. Although currently unemployed, I maintain my self-imposed limits that I set while working as well: I do not touch any until AT LEAST 6 or 7 PM, and that is primarily to relax, relieve pain, and allow me to eat. I am not a 'stoner'. I didn't smoke from the age of 21 until about 35, when I decided to give it a try for the pain and bad stress/anxiety, and it worked wonders so I've stayed with it. Approximated amounts about how much I smoke since I always use hash oils in vaporizer pens and rarely 'smoke' marijuana in

leaf form. I do NOT get any relief from any edibles, no matter how strong or how much I eat.

486. I have a strong understanding that the use of Cannabis should be regulated to that of medical use for minors but should be completely legalized for use in any for by adults. I see no negative results in my self and I see no reason it shoulf not be responsibly used by adults. Thank you for your study.

487. I have adult-onset epilepsy. I started having tonic-clonic seizures when I was 23 and no one knows why. I used to be on prescription anti-epileptic drugs and they helped but they had bad side effects and I still had seizures occasionally. On the recommendation of my neurologist, I decided to give medical cannabis a try. Here's my experience: An edible form of hash oil like Rick Simpson oil seems to work best for stopping auras and seizures. Smoked cannabis is somewhat effective, but does not seem to work as well for reducing seizures. I make hash oil myself from buds I buy at the dispensary using this recipe: http://growweedeasy.com/cannabis-extract-hash-oil I get high-CBD strains to make a high-CBD oil, and high-THC strains to make a high-THC oil. I take 3 drops of high-CBD hash oil in the morning, and 3 drops of high-THC hash oil in the evening, and this has allowed me to go off my anti-epileptic drugs (which didn't work well for me anyway - I was still having seizures), which was a slow process under the care of my neurologist. Every medical cannabis strain I've ever tried apparently seems to be effective. It really seems like any strain will work. I'm not sure it's even necessary I use the high-CBD strains. When they are not available, I take high-THC oil for my morning and night dose but I still don't get seizures. But I hear CBD is better for during the day so that's

what I do in the morning when I can. Regarding your driving question - I choose not to drive at all, more because I'm worried about having a seizure while driving than because I believe I'm impaired from the cannabis. After taking the drops every day, I'm not even sure I feel the effects at all any more.

488. I have always been a recreational user, claiming medicinal benefits but never having been diagnosed or prescribed. While I don't believe it to be chemically addictive, I believe it to be habit forming and can have minor withrawl (indicated above). I am very interested in this survey, and would be willing to participate further if needed without anonymous protections. xxxxxxx@gmal.com

489. I have always loved cannabis. I'm a disabled RN with fibromyalgia/IBS/depression/anxiety/PTSD/restless leg syndrome. I'm also an ACTivist for MMJ here in xxx state. I hate taking opiates but I do need them. Using cannabis helps to relax my muscles and improves my mood, which in turn decreases my pain and improves my quality of life. I think patients should have safe access to medical marijuana AND I think it should be legalized for recreational use. I am affiliated with xxxxxxxxxxxxxxxxxxxxxxxxxxxxxxxxxxxxxxxxxxxxxx. I think people need more education and we need to continue research on cannabinoids. Good luck Washington State :)

490. I have an aggressive form of cancer, which has not affected my health so far. I'm not doing any chemo treatments, but have been interested in cannabis as a cancer healer, and might make and use cannabis oil in the event I get to stage 4.

491. I have anxiety and severe panic attacks that started in my early

twenties. I'm fairly sure its genetic from my mothers side. I became addicted to benzodiazepines (prescribed) after taking them for a few years. When I stopped I became housebound. Cannabis helped me with anxiety, loss of appetite, insomnia, depression, and I am able to function without taking SSRIs.

492. I HAVE ANXIOETY BECAUSE OF CHRONIC PAIN,I CAN RELAX MY TMJ-LESS PAIN IN FACE AND NECK

493. I have been a daily cannabis smoker most of my adult life. I do believe it is habit forming and I would considered myself 'habituated' to cannabis. I don't think it is 'addictive' but for me stopping for some period of time is probably a good thing. But I enjoy it so much that it is hard to stop. It may be affecting my life negatively in some way but overall I function normally in the world.

494. I have been a daily smoker for over 20 years. I'm educated, employed, a single mother of 2 and on top of the things in my life. I also am in the midst of a fairly sever depression. I use cannabis to relax after work, to sleep through the night, and to reduce the amount of anxiety about the world around me and my kids on a daily basis. I believe in the effectiveness of herbs that grow freely on the planet, and I mainly use herbs to combat illness in my family & for preventative remedies.

495. I have been a daily user for 30 years I started getting extreme knee pain and when I was unable to score some weed about 4 days out the pain would go away as soon as scored and started smoking the pain came back and the pain was so bad I would wish that my leg would be cut off. I tried this 2 more times with same results.it has gotten to the point were despite me wanting

to continue I feel that I have come to the end of enjoying canibus because the pain in my knee is not worth the high please look into this. I Know that it sounds crazy but no one loves weed more than me and would sure like to continue into my golden years partaking but the pain is that bad to stop me in my tracks I even had x rays done showing nothing is wrong with the knee

496. I have been able to live my life with only moderate depression and anxiety without the use of prescription drugs by medicating with marijuana.

497. I have been an almost daily smoker for 25 years. I have held great jobs and made great salaries and am respected by my peers in my field. Cannabis use has never impacted any of these factors. Im a new father and just about the most responsible human I know. I think that a life with Cannabis is as liveable and valuable as a life without. Its a choice we should be free to make as long as we dont impact or harm others due to our behaviors.

498. I have been diagnosed with Autism Spectrum Disorder (mild).

499. I have been smoking on average about a joint a day for the last 30 years. I will retire in about 3 years with my $160,000.00 house paid for.

500. I have been smoking since I was 18, so 12 years now. Everyday. I love my life, my wife, my cats, my neighbours, and I am successful in my job.

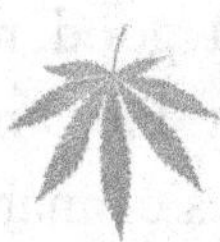

501. I have been smoking weed for 7 years now and have never had a problem with quitting to get a job that required a drug test. When I toke up I feel like my brain is cleared and I can understand things more.

502. I have been through spells of cannabis abuse, and do not deny that it can be abused, but I firmly disbelieve that the substance is in any way, shape, or form, addictive. When I have found cessation of cannabis use difficult, it has invariably been due to my own malaise which I was regulating with cannabis at the time. As soon as the emotional problems are resolved, cessation is immediate and effortless. I also feel that cannabis has helped bolster my immune system, as since I began smoking cannabis regularly, the overall quality of my health has improved. I don't know whether this is directly attributed to the pharmacodynamics of the drug as I feel it is at least in part due to the improvement of mind-body wellness I have experienced as a result of the improvement in my mental health that cannabis has brought about.

503. I have been using cannabis for 8 months and it has helped my anxiety tremendously and has encouraged me to seek therapy for my it. I am 39 years old and never used it as my mother abused prescription drugs, alcohol and cannabis and this put me off. My current partner is a long term user and i asked to try it. He holds down a good well paid job.

504. I have been using cannabis for the past 12-13 years. I was an intercollegiate athlete, I have my masters degree. I am in education, and have a good relationship with my students and staff. Good family life, and good relationship with my girlfriend who also uses cannabis. I am an average individual

that completes my tasks, pays my bills on time, I have an excellent credit score.

505. I have been using cannabis on a recreational basis for 40 years. I can function well in any setting even immediately using it. In my late teens and 20s, I did sometimes try other drugs - cocaine, LSD, MDA. But, I never had a problem with any drugs, including cannabis and alcohol. I rarely drink alcohol - I don't like losing control. With cannabis, I remain in control of myself, my emotions, my actions. I believe that there are medical uses for the plant and wish we could utilize the plant more for that.

506. I have been using cannabis recreationally since the age of 14 everyday use started at the age of 17 I am employed and have always held work I tend to

507. I have been using for the majority of my teenage/young adult years. Your brain is like a muscle;if you don't use it or stretch your limits then you will not improve dexterity. Same with laziness, it is not specifically caused by cannabis, it is just more well pronounced when under the influence.

508. I have chronic back problems due to an accident 18 years ago. They are inoperable and to this point therapy and treatments have not been successful in pain control

509. I have chronic migraines, which is why I use MMJ. They range in frequency from a couple times a month to several times a week, and I have no known triggers. I relied on NSAID pain medication for several years before trying MMJ, partially due to stomach issues (ulcers, etc) that I was worried might be

worsened by NSAID usage. While I won't use MMJ if I have anything important to do for the rest of the day, it provides near instant relief, and I'm hoping that the prophylactic effect my doctor mentioned starts to take effect so I can cut down the number and/or intensity of the migraines. As far as recreational usage goes, I prefer marijuana to alcohol for several reasons. Headaches and hangovers are less common, it has a much less likely chance of negatively affecting my mood, sometimes I get a creative boost, and I feel more lucid when buzzed on weed than I do on alcohol. I have quite a low tolerance for both, but I tend to feel run down after drinking. Marijuana sometimes makes me feel sleepy, but it isn't necessarily a bad feeling. The only other drug I use regularly is caffeine in coffee/tea. I don't drive, and I don't tend to go out while drunk or high because I don't want to find myself in a bad situation.

510. I have chronic upper back neck and shoulder pain due to NERVE damage from a car accident 20 years ago. I worked to support my family for several more years after the injury which didn't help my body any. Then I went from lots of over the counter meds to morphine daily for over the last ten years. I also was diagnosed with fibromyalgia with complications including leaky gut syndrome. After 10 years of narcotics and no improvement I've recently decided to change my approach from pacifing to healing & found a doctor that leans towards holistic meds. To make a long story short I have been able to cut my morphine by 1/3 & during good weather I can reduce it by half! I believe eventually I will be able to manage all of my pain with cannabis, cannabis oils & edibles. It may not ever take away all of the pain but if it makes me be able to garden and play with my grandkids and pushes the pain to the back of my mind then I'm a winner.....I do however, also believe

that this is the best chance I have at possibly HEALING MY NERVE DAMAGE from the accident as well as HEALING MY AUTOIMMUNE SYSTEM.....It's about more than getting 'high' for me. It's a way to be healed.

511. I have experienced acute undiagnosable joint pain and chronic fatigue for 11 years. Nothing else helps, but cannabis takes the edge off. I don't smoke while my children are with me, so my frequency is different than if I was not a half time parent.

512. I have found cannabis to be extremely helpful with the symptoms I have from the Iraq war. The only negative side effect I have found is it's legality.

513. I have found that cannabis use has helped my quality of life with fibromyalgia. I am a closet user due to the stigma of cannabis.

514. I have had 20 years of chronic pain in my neck, shoulders and arms. Cannabis has helped me avoid a depending on over-the-counter pain-reducers like Ibuprofen and Tylenol.

515. I have had many operations, including lumbar back fusion xxxxxxxxxx, which has helped me so much I have only filled my prescription for pain medication 1 time since then (not every month). I have a screw holding my xxxxxxxxx joint together + 2 other xxxxxxxxx surgeries, genetic bone issues & osteoporosis. I am + for HLA - B27, as well as my daughter, who has Cohon's, I have IBS, gastric reflux, hiatal hernia, fybro, 3 xxxxxx surgeries from ACL reattachment xxxxxx, + 1 R knee surgeries xxxx, sleep disorder, cervical spine compression, migraines, no family support. Without my service dog & MMJ I would not be able to cope. I am in therapy, have good surgeons,

trust in God, & hope for my future is more positive since my back fusion & vertebra repair. Edibles help with recovery pain as much as prescriptions. I still need to be strong enough to replace both knees before I get much older, for which I have lots of anxiety about. I also have dormant histoplasmosis so can't take immune suppressing medications, 4 kidney stones (had lithotripsy in 90's for 1 successfully) & 4 nodules on my thyroid, very poor night time vision. I could go on I guess but that's plenty! I don't have money to participate in any activities due to financial issues of chronic illness & its cost. I am very isolated socially for which MMJ helps me cope with as well.

516. I have intractable PTSD; I've done everything from various therapies to psych meds for years, and nothing worked. Cannabis isn't a cure, but it makes the disease manageable enough that I can function pretty normally. I feel that it saved my life.

517. I have lupus and for years was living on pain meds -- vicodin & methadone I have not had any pain meds for 3 years. I have found that eatables work better for my pain and to help me sleep. Why 3 years? because that is when my son made me cannabis chocolate and I have not had a pain pill since! I smoke on occasion for recreational uses but it is mainly for pain relief

518. I have more than 20 years in AA. It was an excruciating decision to start taking cannabis, and I can't talk about it at meetings. But AA friends who knew me before my MS, and my sponsor, helped me understand how to treat it like any other medication.

519. i have ms it makes thing better for me or calms my feelings

520. I have Multiple Sclerosis and 2 stents in my heart. Cannabis definitively helps with all of my MS symptoms and greatly improves my quality of life. Cannabis is my medication of choice to deal with my autoimmune disease. In addition, it helps tremendously in coping with the stress/anxiety/depression which often accompany chronic illness. I have been able to replace several harmful medications (muscle relaxers, pain relievers, etc.) with cannabis, avoiding many harmful and addictive side effects of the pharmaceuticals. The edibles greatly improve spasticity issues. I have never experienced any harmful side effects in my use. I was diagnosed around 31 and am now 61. My friends/acquaintances who chose to use the experimental injections for MS have experienced a much lower quality of life and most are no longer living.

521. I have nerve pain, most likely related to 'severe, complex scoliosis' (physiatrist's diagnosis), which causes vertebra L4 + L5 to press on a nerve root. while cannabis, esp. sativa-dominant, high-THC strains sometimes are very helpful, other times they do nothing, even making things worse (I end up thinking about the pain more) - this could simply be a matter of being distracted by being 'energized' (sativa) high, but I haven't been able to ascertain if that's what's going on. indicas, which dispensaries often recommend for pain, seem less effective on my symptoms. I've also tried high CBD strains, as well as eating raw high CBD/THC strains (to not get high while still getting the analgesic effect), but they didn't work. 'budtenders' - at least the more professional ones, have frequently suggested THC, or THC + CBD, for nerve pain, but it hasn't always worked for me, esp. when the pain is particularly bad, going above '3'. I should mention that I've taken full advantage of the dispensaries, tried over 50 strains, used careful methodology (track dosages, take

notes, repeat the experiment, space out use to avoid building tolerance) - there are clearly (to me at least) major differences between strains as far as analgesic qualities, unrelated to THC/CBD amount differences - some strains really seem more analgesic, with repeat usage confirming initial impressions. given all the strains out there, I'm not planning on attempting to figure out all the better pain-relievers; I've found enough strains that have worked frequently so I can just go back to those. unfortunately, it seems that getting pain relief, for me, means getting high, so if my pain level rises to 4 or 5 or more, and is chronic, that would present me with a difficult choice: be high all the time or hurt. I suppose that if that does happen, and my pain is bad and chronic, I'll really find out if (and/or how well) THC works.

522. I have never had any issue with dependance with this plant. I occasionally smoke it and find it helps significantly with my ADHD symptoms i have never NEEDED to smoke but enjoy it when i do.

523. I have not really tried to go without as I just feel more secure knowing I have access to my medicine whenever I need it. Also, my bi-polar friend is now an alcoholic because his job drug tests making his condition worse. Before when he was able to partake of herb it helped his condition but since he can not he substitutes alcohol, a more harmful substance, for marijuana. We envision the day that MJ will be treated like alcohol nationally especially as it is related to worker's rights.

524. I have only smoked weed about 5 times in my life.

525. I have only used marijuana for a couple years. I use it in place

of prescription pain meds. Way less side effects.

526. I have rarely used it. I first tried it through friends who do it daily. I do it every once in a while. My friends who do it regularly say that it isn't necessarily the cannibus that is addictive, it's more the lifestyle or routine so to say of doing it. I do not like it. It makes me freak out and get really paranoid. Plus if I'm really high I get pretty unsocial and just sit there. And from what I know, it's expensive and it seems very pointless to waste your money on it. But for some people they have different reactions so for them it may be 'worth it.'

527. I have received multiple tickets while high and I would credit it to being unlucky rather than because I was high. Hell, it's happened multiple times and the cops have never noticed any impairment in me. Cannabis is slightly addictive for heavy users although the addiction is extremely easy to overcome compared to other drugs. It's more of a psychological addiction rather than being addicted to the chemicals in the drug. Not everyone experiences the psychological addiction either.

528. I have recently cut back my cannabis use/consumption in hopes to motivate myself to 'do' things more. I went from medicating a few times a day to medicating only a few times a week. I have found that I indeed am more motivated to start projects and be social. I have also lost a significant amount of weight in the past 1.5 months that my use has been limited. Its hard to tell if my weight loss has been from less cannabis or a by product of less cannabis. In any case I have found that though cannabis helps with my chronic pain I am benefiting more from limited use for my daily life function.

529. i have recently stopped taking my anti seizure medication which I took for over 50 years with absolutely no occurance of seizures. I stopped taking the drug over a two year period of time with very small reductions. In the past when I tried to quit I would immediately have a seizure. Now not even a petit seizure.

530. I have reduced mental health medication as well as pain medication by using marijuana under medical supervision. I completely replaced Oxycottin with Marijuana without experiencing any detox symptoms from the oxycottin

531. I have regained a quality of life with medical cannabis that was lost for 20 years while I was on prescriptions for Fibromyalgia.

532. I have seen cannabis improve peoples lives beyond belief, mine included, I have also seen it ruin peoples lives. Just like anything, it is the user not the drug that makes the difference.

533. I have seen someone be on 45 miligrams of THC and she drove. She avoided 3 accidents that weren't her fault in the first place and not once have I heard of someone having an accident while being high. Being high while driving only makes you more careful. You're too lazy and don't care enough to speed.

534. I have Seizures, chronic costochondritis, and severe headaches (that sometimes last for a few days) along with chronic fatigue and random aches & pains. Also anxiety.

535. I have served 4 tours as an infantryman. I have moderate ptsd and moderate myofacial pain in my upper back. I have degenerative discs in my lower back.

536. I have sever ddd and pot is the only that releaves the pain enuff to do the mist common things

537. I have severe IBS symptoms and was only going to the bathroom once a week. No laxative or fiber supplements ever helped. Once I started smoking it completely helped the tightness in my intestines and I was able to go every single day and I always have a good time when I smoke whereas I used to not enjoy some things. I also believe cannabis improved my ability to drive because I am a lot more focused on driving and I am much more careful and less aggressive

538. I have severe reactions to pain meds. I had quit smoking mj for 10 years, then found I needed an alternative to the pain meds. I do not smoke all the time, I use it as a medication. I have stopped for periods of time, yet no withdrawal symptoms at all, unlike the pain meds I had previously been on. MJ does not in any way, get in the way of my quality of life.

539. I have smoked Cannabis for many years now and enjoy it. I have been responsible throughout my life. I have never like drinking alcohol. It makes me mad that I am thought of as a criminal for using Cannabis when in reality I am a good person and cause no harm to society.

540. i have smoked cannabis for over 20 years almost daily until 2 years ago i gave up smoking. i now vaporise once a night every other night or when i want to eat a lot more than i do because im under weight and smoking gives me an appetite so i eat more. i done my driving test and every job interview using cannabis and have been in employment from i left school. i cannot remember the last time i was off sick from work and my boss

tells me i have the best sickness record in my dept for which i have worked for eleven years. i also drove daily using cannabis being very aware of speed limits and road signs, however after stopping smoking and using cannabis daily i think my driving has become more erratic. i have never had an accident driving with cannabis and dont beleive it makes me not people me a worse driver . I also beleive eople have differrent tolerances to cannabis. i liked to smoke skunk which some people dont like hope this helps

541. I have smoked Cannabis since the age of 16, pretty much twice a day, with an occasional interruption due to supply. I smoke an excessive amount of tobacco, and have for many years. Cancer runs in my family, yet I have not had it. I attribute that to Cannabis. Further, I have extreme arthritis, which is kept in check by Cannabis. I do a physical labor job, and while I find myself slowing down as I age, I can continue to work because of Cannabis.

542. I have smoked pot since I was 19 in 1965. I was/am an alcoholic but quit drinking in 1975 at age 29. Pot was never anything like alcohol, ever in any way. I have always driven after smoking or during driving. I like it still at 67. I think I'm getting a bit old for this but still doing it. One thing though is I live in a very rural place without traffic of much kind. I doubt I could smoke and drive in a city or on a busy LA freeway. I could but it wouldn't be smart. No tickets, no accidents but a couple coulda been problems. I was a serious danger when I drank. I have no children and have started three businesses of which one is still operating after 35 years. People tell us all the time we have the best xxxx shop ever. I'm in Rotary, I was xxxxxxxxxxxxxxxx Citizen of the Year, Chamber of commerce etc. every kind of

person smokes pot. I live in xxxxxxxxxxxxxxxxxxxxxxxxx so I live in the right place to make it easy. After almost fifty years of daily use...two to three joints a day.....I am happy to be part of any study. xxxxxxxxxxxxxxx

543. I have smoked recreational for years, but I always knew it calmed me and my hyperactive personality, it made me a calmer parent, when I stopped fro 5 years my pain became out of control, I became addicted to opoids during that time, with the assistance of the medical marijuana commuity I removed myself from all prescription medications and have found that different types of cannabis have easily taken the place of these meds, I now have my life back with my family and I am now enjoying grandchildren that I thought I'd never see... it's a wonderful plant and it's natural, should also note I smoked for all three of my pregnancies and gave birth to three health children who are now healthy adults with healthy children

544. I have smoked since 1967, at age 24. I smoke daily now. I have never found smoking to be deleterious to my health. my biggest concern has always been obtaining it because it is illegal. and, of course, worrying that I might get 'nabbed' for possessing it. I now do the most logical thing. I grow my own. no drug deals, no money for cartels, and I am certain what the product is. the war on drugs will go down as one of the biggest boondoggles ever promulgated by the us government. it's only a matter of time before it becomes legal, and its countless benefits will be found true through research.

545. I have substituted cannabis with alcohol. I use cannabis for intractable pain.

546. I have suffered from PTSD and bipolar depression for over 10 years.

547. I have suffered many tragedy's in life and depression with bipolar disease I have taken all kinds of meds but nothing has ever worked, the first time I smoked was age 13 and not again till 16 then on and off in high school then just every once in awhile till age 28 then quite a bit but since age 38 every day or almost every day I take no drugs at all at the present and haven't in years the only thing I use is cannabis and I really can tell a difference on my depressions and over all mental health is much more improved!

548. I have suffered with depression and I've found that sativa dominant strains help me feel more cheerful and I am an artist as well and cannabis does help get the creative juices flowing as well. I wish I could be a medical patient but I have just not taken the time to actively go out and obtain one.

549. I have used cannabis medicinally for 40 years. When I was about 35, I was forced to stop my therapy for 5 years. It was very detrimental to my health. I shortly required pharmaceutical meds for blood pressure and began a journey into Hell. By 51, with failing health, forced to retire and at 53 told I had 6 months to live. Got off 22 meds, 9 surgeries, lost 200 lbs. and got 4 titanium joints. Last hip total replacement under general, cannabis oral and topical, with 4 Norco's and went home day one post op. Able to decrees doses when able to vaporize and smoke at home. I have learned through cannabis therapy the importance of holistic medicine, including acupuncture, physical and occupational therapy, and meditation with positive visualization. I am limited physically(96% total

disability/ workman's comp) but cannabis gives me clarity of mind. Having gone so close to death, I want to live fully and cannabis, in all its forms has been a true blessing. Compared to my life in 2003, I am truly living my dreams. Thank you cannabis for the improvement. Not easy but when balanced in with activity, diet, and auxiliary treatments I have found peace of mind.

550. I have used cannabis medicinally since 2011 and study my own use to manage a neurological/spinal disorder that I have had since age 9. I get my best results for pain from raw cannabis and topicals. I make my own medibles to avoid foods that I am sensitive to (gluten, dairy, sugar, eggs, corn, rice, soy.) I chronicle my cannabis findings, adventures, and recipes at xxx xxxxxxxxxxxxxxxxxxxxxxxxxxxxxx.

551. I have used cannabis since I was young. I have never had a bad experience with it and it's done nothing but positive things for me. I come from a past of a lot of trauma and abuse, I will be the first to say that cannabis helps me feel better and makes life feel more positive and peaceful for me as a person. I would live everyday, all day on cannabis if I were able to. It makes me less anxious and feel like a better person. Depending on the strain, it gives me more motivation to get up and do stuff, helps me worry less, calms my racing thoughts down, etc. I also feel like it helps me be a more peaceful and thoughtful mother. These are just my experiences though. :) I use it for menses as well.

552. I have used cannabis to relax my muscle spasms in my back, in which these spasms have caused bulging discs and loss of nerves/reflexes in my legs. I also prefer cannabis to alcohol due to the effects of alcohol such as not being able to drive at all

(when I use cannabis I drive like a grandma) and hangovers.

553. I have used for quite some time, there have been periods of heavier usage. In my late teens, I would smoke around 20 grams a week. Most of the time there has been periods of use of about 2-4 g a week for several months, followed by several months of usuage closer to a gram a month. In CA, I was given medical license, but have not at my new location.

554. I haven't smoked/ate Cannabis in years because it would put me to sleep. I have been hearing about the Cannabis now that will help with fatigue and spasms. I have tried edibles and it helped but not as well as smoking it. Also I used a dot, I think they call it tincture, I have some messed up dreams and will NEVER use that again. With smoking it I tried one type and it didn't help at all, then I tried another type that made me feel awake. I don't want to smoke it so I haven't been doing it. I also don't like that the shops cannot tell you that what it is and what is in it.

555. i hope this helps legalize cannabis in the near future so our government can stop wasting time money and resources on the most medically/spiritually/industrially beneficial plant in existence.

556. I hope this helps.

557. I just had to take a piss test for a job with a headquarters outside of California. Even though I have a medical recommendation, I may not get the job if Marijuana is found in my urine.

558. I just like to use cannabis to relax and reward myself for

studying all day since I'm a medical student. I'm doing a thesis paper on medical cannabis later this year and am excited to get researching. Good luck!

559. I just want to say I have arrived DOA on three occassions due to prescription pain killers. They are killers alright...marijuana is safer.

560. I know marijuana helps with my overall quality of life.

561. I like it and its the only law I break.

562. I like turtles

563. I live in CT. We could use any help we can get too.

564. I live in Germany where beer is equal to water and marijuana to heroin. I drink beer and liquor only on weekends but I take cannabis allmost every day but only before sleep. I also never drive under the influence of cannabis. Getting special sorts of marijuana(see the point with the selection of mmj) is very hard, I just take what comes, but in the selection I choose what I would take if I had the opportunity. I hope I could help.

565. I lost 4 years out of my life due to pharmaceuticals cannabis has given me my life back and I am now pharmaceutical free

566. I love cannabis and consider it the most effective form of natural medicine

567. I love cannabis, it really helps me relieve anxiety and improve my creativity for work. I don't believe cannabis is addictive,

but when I haven't been using it, it's hard for me to have an appetite.

568. i love cannabis.keep on doing what you are doing :)

569. I love it but besides recreational it should be used medicinally and for manufacturing

570. I love it but don't abuse it

571. I love marijuana very much and I will continue to use it no matter what the laws say. By decriminalizing it's use I won't have to go to a dodgy dealer in a dodgy dangerous part of town to get it. I will also know exactly what I am buying, currently the product I get can be laced with other substances to make cheap weed stronger. The money I spend might found other crime at the moment, if I could buy it from a trusted source I know where the money is going or I can just save money and grow my own weed (which at the moment is very difficult because owning plants is illegal and could lead to hefty fines or jail time). There are many positives to decriminalization and seemingly not much change in terms of what people think are 'negatives'

572. I love the smell of cannabis plants but hate the taste. I have mainly (in 7 months with med auth) used edibles and concentrates like Mount Siarlequin capsules sublingually.

573. I love weed

574. I love weed!

575. I make a topical cannabis liniment that kills the pain of gallstones, broken bones, bone spurs, arthritis, headaches, sprains, bunions, sore muscles. The hospital wants to give me demerol for gallstone and my liniment works better. The only thing that prevents nausea in me is my first bite of food in the am is cannabis infused. Without it I am nauseous. Alcohol make me sick, cannabis relaxes me.

576. I make edibles for MS and Cancer patients and I believe it is a very potent effective herb that cures and certainly helps most human ailments. Not only is it fun to use recreationally, it is healing and rejuvenating.

577. I marked boxes that contradict each other because I can concentrate better after cannabis use on creative endeavors, like music dancing art, but concentrate less on reading and learning new things. I only have anxiety if I smoke too much.

578. I most use cbd oil now and smoke cannabis much less. The cbd oil I take daily has changed my life in a profound way! It has almost eliminated symtoms from several health problems I have. It makes me feel like my mind, body and soul are in perfect synch and at peace. I can function highly in life whereas before my symptoms prevented me from doing so.

579. I never could understand smoking cannabis because it never did the same thing twice & was uncomfortable as a minor when people kept pressuring with it always coming around. I thought those that used cannabis for even arthritis, which I have a very severe form of (ankylosing spondylitis-autoimmune disorder), were using it to smoke to get high to forget the pain a little while & I was against that. Now I found

out it has slowed the activity of the disease & cures cancers; yet I have an autoimmune disorder that reacts to substances very differently than others. Medical Cannabis my opportunity to see if it will assist this autoimmune disorder & shrink large nodular densities in both breasts needing surgery, which I have refused to do Rick Simpson Oil (RSO) instead. It has only been 2 weeks of trying to get used to the RSO, it is hard, but I am willing to keep trying. The autoimmune disorder has worsened a little as our weather got worse, but I am sticking with this to help others in case there is a good outcome. It hurts a lot so I hope I can stay on RSO & get the benefits of it.

580. I never tried cannabis prior to turning 21 as I believed it was as bad as other illegal drugs. I witnessed my friends smoking cannabis recreationally. I tried cannabis for the first time then and felt that it was a healthier recreational choice for my body/mind than alcohol, since social drinking always made me ill. I never drank alcohol again after discovering recreational cannabis. Shortly after becoming a recreational user I came to a realization that cannabis was bringing me significant relief from digestive issues, extreme case of insomnia and symptoms of psychological distress. I have since continued to use cannabis medicinally whenever possible as it is the safest medicine and the most effective that I currently know of to help me get a good nights sleep. My digestive issues (diagnosed IBS) and my symptoms of psychological distress (highly sensitive person, PTSD, anxiety) are grossly exacerbated when I am unable to sleep at night. I find the cost of cannabis to be extremely prohibitive(in addition to the laws) so there have been periodic times I have suffered more having to abstain for legal or work purposes or inability to afford the herb.

581. I never used recreational drugs when at university in the 60s and gave up drinking alcohol. I think it is important to separate information about medical cannabis from negativity of recreational use. This is even though I see cannabis doing less harm than opiates, alcohol, tobacco. For me it is like a magic wand - the pain decreases so quickly and so markedly and the relief last hours. I am hoping MC will soon be available in Australia and would be happy to complete further surveys.

582. I often self-medicate while on my period.

583. I only achieve my desired relief when I have access to California's system periodically. I have held a card there for four years and I need access to a variety of strong meds for different activities as well as sleep and pain relief.

584. I only like smoking; ingesting does not work for me, but I am also curious about new products as well as learning more about/ having choices of strains

585. I only recently tried cannabis after 38 years because it is legal in Washington now. I did not like it because I could not feel spirit. I went for a walk in the forest and found my connection with nature was diminished. I remember my youthful use of cannabis and alcohol and other drugs and never want to be in that place again. I will never use it again.

586. I only use cannabis at night, when all chores are finished because I get easily distracted by random thoughts when stoned

587. I only use Cannabis if someone offers it at a club or party, so I rarely use it.

588. I only use salves and oils topically, preferably with low yo no THC because I don't like to feel high. I don't smoke pot because it hurts my lungs. I have chronic pain due to scar tissue and arthritis in my spine from injuries. I use marijuana and movement therapy. If I did not I would not be able to move

589. I personally believe that it's impossible to forge a physical dependency on cannabis. I can and have gone a month or two without with no form of physical craving. This is even more powerful when you take into account that I am and have been a very heavy cannabis user over the past few years. Cannabis helps you explore your own subconscious, what could be more liberating than that? p.s. The only reason I've got negative attributes i.e paranoia for what I feel when I stoned is due to weed I've smoked in England. Weed I've smoked while in Amsterdam and California have given me no negative side effects. Most likely due to them being heavily regulated and being grown in laboratory conditions.

590. I personally feel cannabis has overall improved my well being. Yes, there are some drawbacks. But, it's the best medicine I use to help my anxiety.

591. I personally have never heard of anyone close to me having issues with driving or becoming addicted to cannabis. That being said, I don't think that it is impossible or that there have not been cases of people becoming addicted or driving poorly. I also believe that there are potential negative impacts on the undeveloped mind and should be used cautiously. Like nearly everything in life, cannabis should be used in moderation and definitely not for escapism or as a social lubricant.

592. I personally use cannabis to help me eat before every meal I use it to keep myself focused at work and other activities also it makes me more sociable and creative helps me relax gets rid of my back pain temporarily (usually a couple hours) also to help me sleep at night

593. I personally use it mostly at night, before bed, as pain management and a sleep aide. I do enjoy how it makes me feel, however, and will regularly take breaks from it every month or so, even though it's difficult to do so.

594. I prefer Cannabis over Adderall for my ADHD.Cannabis works way better and with no side effects.

595. I prefer cannabis over prescription for chronic pain management. I also use recreationally and prefer it over alcohol, although I am a light to moderate drinker. I usually don't mix the two.

596. I prefer to vaporize because of asthma.

597. I primarily vape at night to help tolerate neck and shoulder pain and stiffness due to poor posture and sitting at computer all day.

598. I put that I don't think Cannabis is addictive, but for some people it can certainly be addictive. I feel like a lot of people use it habitually though. Not necessarily addicted but still using it consistently.

599. I quit alcohol years ago but every once in awhile a little toke of pot helps to take the edge off, I still feel like I have to hide the fact that I smoke every now and then but that it is perfectly

acceptable for people to have a beer or a glass of wine to unwind. Not everyone is a hard core pot smoker.

600. I rarely use cannabis 'recreationally'. I use it as a medicine. Sometimes my friends and I share :)

601. I really appreciate that you are doing these surveys to get honest, anonymous opinions from cannabis users. I hope more universities start researching it and find the positive aspects of cannabis use. Thank you

602. I really think it should be legal, nation-wide. The fact that I have to be a criminal to experience pain relief is ridiculous.

603. I recently cut down on my use from multiple times a day for the past 5 years to roughly 2-3 a month (~1-2 hits/session). All of the above information is heavily dependent on set and setting for me and I make a conscious effort to not necessarily use cannabis as a cure for any personal issues.

604. I recently moved to a part of the country where the penalty for possession is very stiff so I haven't been using Cannabis to treat my conditions aside from during infrequent visits to my city of origin. I accomplish in a month what I used to accomplish in a few days when I used it daily. If the opportunity arises, I will be moving somewhere that I can get a medical card. The effect on my inflammation and anxiety especially improves my quality of life immensely. Thank you for doing this study.

605. I rediscovered marijuana once it became legal. I have been surprised by some of the positive effects of vaporizing about an eighth of a teaspoon a few times a week. It has helped with

many perimenopausal issues, such as helping me to sleep better, evening out my moods and reducing anxiety. I feel it has also helped me have a greater appreciation for the arts and creativity in general. And I think I am even a better parent. I did have a bit of a learning curve with it at first. I started using it when it became legal more on a whim, recreational. But now I really appreciate the wellness aspects.

606. I resent that it is illegal, difficult. & expensive to obtain; I think growing your own in small quantities should be legal; research on its use in managing anxiety would be helpful- I.e., does it promote increased alpha waves on EEG? Thank you for your work in this area!

607. I say cannabis is not addictive, but that isn't entirely true. I think discontinuation symptoms occur and cannabis improves many common ailments like fatigue, poor mood, and aches and pains. When people stop using cannabis, they go back to feeling worse than they did on cannabis. Some doctors and scientists describe this as addiction but the degree of addiction to things like nicotine or alcohol are substantially worse. To those that say cannabis is addictive as an argument against its use, I use the example of a person who benefits from prescription medication- is this person addicted in the same way you would say someone is addicted to marijuana?

608. I select my strains by trial and error then use what works for pain relief. Other varieties are used recreationally and to look for pain relief alternatives.

609. I selected a few answers that are polar opposites in the same section because depending on the strain my motivation and energy can be wildly different.

610. I smoke a little after work. Nice way to destress and spend time with my fiancÃ©.

611. I smoke about .5 oz/week. There was no option for that in the survey

612. I smoke before bed so I barely ever dream anymore

613. I smoke marijuana because I enjoy it. although I would have a difficult time turning it down while it's being offered, it has never bothered me to not have it. thus I cannot say for sure if I am addicted or not. if I have it, I smoke it till it's gone. if I don't have it, I go get some, If I cannot get more, it does not bother me and I don't get irritable without it..

614. I smoke only high cbd/very low thc cannabis for pain relief. Since starting the cannabis I have been able to stop taking prescription pain relief meds. I'm pain free & able to function in ways I haven't functioned for 10 years. I'm starting to grow my own now since the cost in the dispensaries is so high.

615. I smoke small amounts of cannabis in the evenings to help calm down/de-stress. It works better than alcohol and has fewer side effects. I may be an alcoholic otherwise.

616. I smoked cannabis in small amounts through both of my pregnancies and during labour for my home birth. Both my children are healthy with no allergies or disorders. They also both gained entry to grammar schools without any tutoring for the exam and my daughter attends the 3rd best grammar school in the country.The benefits and uses of cannabis are well documented and clearly thats why it remains illegal in the UK.

617. I smoked cannabis regularly while pregnant with my second child. I did so to deal with the horrific nausea I had during my entire pregnancy. My second child is now two years old. He exceeds his older brother (who is five years old) in communication skills (vocabulary) and he has an exceptional memory for books and music. He will certainly be an early reader.

618. I smoked cannabis the entire time I was pregnant.

619. I smoked recreationally wen younger now for medical reasons

620. I started off smoking cannabis when I was 17 as a social thing really, purely recreational. It wasn't until I was in my mid 20's that I started to find the pain relief benefits from it, as I suffered from a bad back. It was the best way to relax my muscles and allow me to stretch and exercise without pain. Then I started using it to help me sleep, as I had endless nights where I'd go without. To this day, I use it both recreationally AND medically (self prescribed) even though it is still 100% illegal where I live.

621. I started to use cannabis in 1969 at age 21. I used for a few years, then stopped for about 15 years. For the past 27 years I have used it nearly every day. During that time I raised three kids and got a college degree with a 3.5 average while working as a mail carrier. I don't think I could have done it without cannabis. Now at age 65 my health is good and I lead an active life. I have a genetic autoimmune disease, but I'm managing it with 100 mg. of Zoloft a day and cannabis. I don't take any other medicines.

622. I started using cannabis again last year as my partner has

cancer and wanted to try it. We were able to procure leaf from xxxxxxxxxxx variety with high THC and Moderate CBD. We tincture it on ice to decrease activation of THC, neither of us want to get high. We use about an ounce of tincture a week. We tincture with 80% alcohol, combo vodka and everclear and water for 4-6 weeks in the freezer. I love the way it tastes and feels. I have found that my sugar cravings decrease when I take it. I don't take it with in 24 hrs before I work (xxxxxxxxxx doctor). My partner has been taking it for almost a year and feels that the lymphoma is not spreading, she is not and has not done any conventional treatment exc one chemo treatment with xxxxxxxxxxxxxxxxx. Felt like she was going to die, stopped treatment, uses only alternative care. Homeopathy, acupuncture, naturopathic medicine. Thanks for your interest.

623. I still enjoy alcohol but when consume cannabis I tend to enjoy the quality of one or maybe two beers rather than drink 4-5. My career is managing office and some days are really stressful so when I get home I don't still want to be stressed so I smoke a bowl or two or half a joint it literally takes the edge off and I go about my night. I feel that cannabis naturally helps me be more connected to the world. Not only has cannabis opened my eyes to the fact that a lot of people have trouble opening up and allowing themselves to be who they truly are, it has also helped me allow myself to be whatever it is that I am. I'm starting to love people I used to loathe. I hope I don't sound out of touch because I feel quite the opposite. Thanks for the opportunity.

624. I stopped using cannabis as a teenager but 32 years later at the age of 50 I was diagnosed with TMJ. I sought medical advice, obtained a recommendation and legally purchased cannabis 4 years ago at the age of 50. Since then my wife and I have had

cannabis around us in tincture form and topical treatments. I grow my own cannabis but often purchase varieties to learn more and to share with others. Since I have begin taking cannabis my overall quality of life has improved. My mood has improved and my relationships at work have improved. I am making the most money I have ever made and I have the most responsibility I have ever had in my professional life. I have begin to play a musical instrument for the first time in my life. I love having a little cannabis every few days and I don't see anything wrong with it.

625. I suffer from bad stomach aches and it helps me ease the stress from them however the reason I use it is still recreational and the relief from the stomach aches is an added bonus

626. I suffer from chemical sensitivity, most petroleum based: gasoline, perfumes, hairsprays, colognes. Not so much nowadays since I'm in a situation where I can avoid exposure. Dunno how the mj fits in, but sometimes I need to laugh, and it helps. Also, I like to toke before physical exercise.

627. I suffer from Chronic pelvic pain & an overactive bladder, and am on medication to treat them. Cannabis aids me more than any medication I am on, and allows me to be pain free for the time it lasts. I frequently stop smoking for weeks at a time and have no withdrawal symptoms. The use of cannabis has increased my quality of life immensely.

628. I suffered from frequent, severe migraines, about once a month, before I started using cannabis. Since I began regularly smoking cannabis 8 years ago, I have only had 5 migraines.

629. I take very low dose orally only. 16mgs per capsule. 1-2x /day 6 hrs in between doses. I've taken rheumatologist prescribed major pain relievers for many yrs. I was shocked to find marijuana taken orally, resin, oil, powdered capsules etc. that's high in CBD very low THC, to have almost the same effect as narcotic pain rx's in it's reduction of the pain and increase of comfort. PTSD sleep trouble relieved by taking Mj at bedtime. I need my brain to work and prefer the very low THC type. I have used it at times to make art, enjoy a walk... I would like the Hi CBD low THC medical use types to be cheaper for people with illness'.

630. I take Zoloft for depression and anxiety. MJ greatly reduces the side effects. I also have some inflammation issues (my lungs swell up, making breathing more difficult) which has gone away since regularly using MJ.

631. I think Cannabis can be addictive; although, I would say majority of the time that it is not addictive and can be stopped. It is a social thing for me sometimes, but there are days when I don't want to be high for whatever reason. Getting medical cannabis was a big deal for me because of how stigmatized it has been while I grew up. But getting off all the above prescription drugs was a way better deal and changed my life for the better! I can sleep when I please now and I do not feel like a zombie roaming the world helplessly. The anti-psychotics that I was previously on only made me more psychotic and on edge, even attempted suicide a few times while on those drugs. Since I started using cannabis there has been no turning back. I made straight A's in college and got accepted into a medical program to become a doctor. I think cannabis affects everyone differently just like any mind-altering substance.

632. I think cannabis has medical uses but I also think people tend to abuse the medical excuse.

633. I Think Cannabis Is A God Given Miracle And It Does So Much Good If They would Just Let It!! I Would Soon To Take Something Natural And From The Earth Then Man Made Any Day For My Pain And Depression

634. I think cannabis is addictive, in some ways. Maybe not physically, but you get mentally addicted to it, it's become the only thing me and my friends know how to do together.

635. I think cannabis is an absolute miracle.

636. I think Cannabis is FAR less harmful to society than alcohol. If I were forced to choose between alcohol and cannabis I would certainly choose cannabis. No one goes home and commits an act of domestic violence after smoking a joint!! But many acts of domestic violence result after drinking by the attacker.

637. I think cannabis is great for medicinal purposes and recreational purposes. I believe the culture around cannabis is what has given it such a bad rap. I do however believe that like any substance it can be very addicting and should be used with caution.

638. I think cannabis is only phisical addictive there is no real addictive agents in the bud itself but people become dependent on the effects it creates

639. I think cannabis is psychologically addictive, you like the state it puts you in and that's why you continue use. One of

the greatest benefits of cannabis legalization besides medicinal use is as a raw material (hemp) Everyone should know how much cannabis use is good for them and realize when they are abusing the substance. Its all about balance (golden mean), for me that is use on weekends and ocasionally during the week.

640. I think cannabis is very poorly understood. It isn't until you regularly smoke weed that you begin to benefit the most from cannabis. If you smoke seldom you will get very high, the more you smoke a tolerance will build up. It is once you have a tolerance that you are able to enjoy your experience. I am excited for the future because I think there are many medical benefits that have not yet been fully proved by science that will be discovered within the next ten years.

641. I think cannabis purchased illegally is much more dangerous. The THC/CBD balance is often much higher on the THC end, which has shown to increase hallucinations and paranoia in those already prone to such states (like Schizophrenics, bipolar, manic, etc.) If we could have legal cannabis it would be so much safer. My spouse uses only high CBD bud because she is prone to such hallucinations. Right now, purchasing cannabis illegally is like going to one of those parties teenagers (unfortunately) have, where you put all the prescription pills in a bag and just grab some and swallow. It's dangerous. Cannabis is truly a great medicine - and one I believe CAN be used recreationally as well as medicinally - and I hope someday we'll be able to use it as such.

642. I think cannabis should be readly available for anyone over the age of 21. I feel like it should be legalized recreationally for everyone. It hurts no one, and helps many. –xxxx

643. I think cannabis use varies a lot depending on the persons sober mental health, past drug use, and overall state of well-being. Degree of usage per smoke session also makes a huge difference on how one might feel throught the 'high', affecting that person differently everytime.

644. i think cannadis is the best drug on the earth in fact its not a drug it is a herb why make something illegal that nature has given use cars kill more than cannabis ever plastic spoons kill more than cannabis

645. I THINK CBD RICH CANNABIS IS FABULOUS, I DON'T FORGET AS MUCH AND FEEL MOTIVATED AND SOOTHED WITH LESS PARANOIA. I PRESENTLY USE A HIGH CBD STRAIN WHICH ALSO HAS SOME THC

646. I think I am a more healthy person due to my cannabis use.

647. I think I'm not as mentally sharp when I smoke weed regularly. Also I'm concerned about the effect on my lungs.

648. I think if it's been longer on the earth than humans or on earth for just as long, not sure of the exact earliest historical contexts but I think it's safe to say it's okay for us.

649. I think if marihuana was legalized or decriminalized that the economic systems would boost. Tax revenues would be 1m plus. Considering all the advancements we are seeing who knows what will come out of cbd We need marijuana legal

650. I think it helps me when I'm in pain I would recommend over a pill any day

651. I think it is a wonderful alternative to increased alcohol intake and can be a great social activity to unwind and relax. Medically, it is an amazing herb that can be useful in so many forms, especially in oil format for those with longstanding, debilitating disease.

652. I think it should be legal in all states. I think we need to be aware of what chemicals are add to it.

653. I think it should be legal never hurts my pyshically I don't know anyone that has OD on it

654. I think it should have been used all along for medical conditions that have now been proven to help. Our pharmaceutical companies are to blame along with the government. Please keep fighting for it and please work to keep the pharmaceutical companies from taking it over they will ruin it.

655. I think it's a great drug that, from what I've seen, effects each user uniquely but generally out of my circles of friends, the ones who are frequent cannabis users have some of the best health and fitness (work out, run, play sports, etc), and overall satisfaction with their lives. They also seem to do well with school and at work, along with being adept socially.

656. I think it's addicting because I get used to it. Use is somewhat sporadic because of lack of availability and funds. I enjoy it, but see it as 'medicine'. If you're not sick, don't need medicine. It helps with PTSD, but I would like to get healed to the point where I no longer need or desire the medicine. I wish it was legal so it would be easy and affordable to acquire. Most people I know grow clones in pots---not nearly as good as the buds 30

yrs ago that we're grown in the earth, from seeds...

657. I think marijuana can be addictive in varying degrees in different people. It is milder to take a few days off of smoking than caffeine in my experience. my alcohol use has been reduced from 1-2 a day and I feel healthier. I am more confident in interacting with others even while un-medicated.

658. I think marijuana should have nutrition labels with thc content and other important things people should know. I would like to thank you for all your efforts to help legalize marijuana!

659. I think people should be allowed to smoke marijuana recreationally. I had surgery for appendicitis last year and enjoyed marijuana as a painkiller, also. My surgeon told me he would rather see me smoke marijuana than drink alcohol.

660. I think perhaps the biggest mistake made by Western Medicine is considering the 'intoxication' provided by cannabis as an unwanted side effect.

661. I think regulation of the quality and purity of Cannabis is the answer. I think it should be legal to recreationally use Cannabis in my state.

662. I think that cannabis has helped me get through life from the day a first tried it . When a was a teenager it kept me away from hard drugs and kept me out of trouble as you are more laid back when stoned. As am forty now and hardly ever been to the doctors apart from problems I had when I used to drink about five years ago . I gave up drinking witch was helped very much by smoking grass , now a only drink in very small doses.

I find through the years I love this shit even more with all the new strains coming on the market . I used to like a drink but price increase kinda put a damper on it so I still smoke and live happy and healthy ...for now anyway

663. I think that Cannabis is a beneficial and enjoyable substance when used and regulated correctly. I think that we could benefit from further legalization and research. I am really looking forward to the legalization in WA state and the increasing acceptance of Cannabis in mainstream culture.

664. I think that cannabis is addictive to some people just like some people become addicted to food, it really depends on the individual and their mental health state

665. I think that many people experience cannabis differently. When I first started i was more creative it didn't affect me in any other aspect of my social life or my mood, however it wasn't until after around 2 years of heavy use that it began affecting my life negatively. So I don't think you can group its effects as other drugs would because there are so many varieties with different effects, I find that sometimes It will give me more motivation and sometimes I become lazy and unmotivated, sometimes I wake up the next day and feel fresh and energized sometimes I wale up and feel groggy and hungover.

666. I think that most of questions tend to be focused on addiction. I know why, but l only wish that folks who were working on Opioids were as focused on the welfare of their patients in this area, as Bastyr is on Cannabis. There are those of us using this for which there isn't a lot of allopathic medicine isn't working well for (such as Dravet's Syndrome, Cerebral Palsy,

Diverticulitis, as well Fibromyalgia). I find it frustrating that most of the focus with cannabis seems to be on the 'reefer madness' level and less on the therapeutic concerns. There was a child who died because the cannabis oil he received was somehow compromised (there wasn't enough oil, or the oil was wrong in dosing, certainly didn't have enough THC to CBD for entourage delivery). When patients or parents of patients cannot talk to their physicians about cannabis, cannabis dosing, or even talk about dual medicine use (allopathic with cannabis), I am not surprised this is happening to patients. Dispensaries are no place to take serious medical usage nor should they be determining plant use (there are plenty of stories by those who work in the industry, claiming that because strain 'A' is considered top shelf, and they have far too much of strain 'B',(which is cheaper, type of cannabis), they tend to stuff the strain 'A' container with strain 'B' product. It's very disconcerting, especially when the need of the patient is specific, not just 'antidotal' . Cannabis needs to be studied seriously, and so does the need for it to be managed medically need to be taken seriously. No family should have to bury their child because the quality of product/care is compromised by greed. When no one is dispensing this by folks with medical training, its a wonder there hasn't been more problems. My parents started taking me to Dr. xxxxxxxxxx, back in 1970, I believe, when Naturopathic medicine was approved for treatment of patients in Washington State. Prior to that, my family took me to Vancouver CN for care in 1967-1969, after an allopathic doctor wanted to give me steroid cream for my female areas following Scarlett Fever. I am stating all this in hopes that Bastyr college members realize that there are a good majority of cannabis users are also inline with homeopathic medicine as well as naturopathic care. The bigger focus in my mind should really be on working on the whole of the plant and how it works, rather than on the questions of 'goofiness', or the focus on recreational concerns, but that's my concern, just as finding out more about the endocannabinoid system (in humans) would be a good thing, since Echinacea and other plants also seem to follow on this pathway.

667. I think that the long term effects of Cannabis use is less addictive and damaging to your system than many of the over the counter and/or prescribed drugs our country and world consumes.

668. I think that weed is not addicting, but when it becomes a daily habit and a lifestyle it is hard to quit and you have withdrawls. I love smoking weed, but if I needed to stop I could cold turkey today. The addiction questions would be better answered by this answer than what I put in the survey.

669. I think the biggest negatives associated with Cannabis are due to it being illegal.

670. I think the fact that it is illegal to smoke cannabis is what causes some people to become paranoid from smoking weed.

671. I think the substance itself its the habits form from the use. People do not like change.

672. I think there are people who can easily become addicted and others who don't have any trouble with it, like anything, alcohol, sugar, exercise....I think making medical grade available at pharmacies, as any other prescription would greatly improve the system of distribution and product regulation.

673. I think there should be a servey comparing those who drink, smoke, or just do one or the other. I personally do both but I don't bindge drink because my mental state can't handle drinking large amounts like most my age. I am judged by most for choosing to smoke instead of drink even though it's safer for me.

674. I think there should be better wording with the question regarding if its addicting. Cannabis is not physically addicting, but many people get confused about their habitual addictions. I appreciate this survey though, very well done

675. I think this is very important research, thank you for conducting it. I also really appreciate your use of the word Cannabis and not Marijuana.

676. I think tracking the side effects of long term use is interesting and important, especially with people whose brains are not fully developed when they start. I also think it would be important to explore the emotional/psychological trends in people with long term use, as well as there level of cognitive ability. I think that my brain function and my emotional/psychological well being have been compromised by long term marijuana use... especially memory, decision making, anxiety, depression... difficulty learning....

677. I think what people see as withdrawals are actually the symptoms from their condition. If you have anxiety or are in pain what ever it maybe you are going to see the body react to not being medicated. What you see is what they would be like all the time without the cannabis.

678. I think with prolonged use you can become addicted to anything, marijuana, food, sex. I believe 100% that it needs to be further studied, but has lots of medical uses and should be reclassified federally. The continued class 1 schedule drug does not fit it. In xxxxxxx, Washington where I live heroin is an issue, meth is an issue, I have never tried or desired to try them. I have been offered other drugs, such as cocaine but I always declined because I had strong personal beliefs about drugs and alcohol, especially because of there correlation with violence. I lost both of my parents at a young age. Alcohol and drugs (crack cocaine) their addictive qualities, and their effects on personality and the choices we make. I was a cigarette smoker for longer than I used cannabis. Recently quit cold turkey by choice even though my husband wasn't quite ready yet. Marijuana is only a gateway drug because of the people you come into contact with trying to get marijuana, if it was decriminalized on a large scale and you didn't buy it from your local neighborhood drug dealer you would not come in contact with other recreational drugs. I think it would lower use in adolescents if we legalized it and we would also lower prison population and arrest rates with legalization or decriminalizing it. I wish it was approved medically in more states. My brother in Minnesota would greatly benefit from medical marijuana for his pain following a serious accident that left him as a quadriplegic. The governor of Minnesota has vetoed it's bills passing even with over 80% approval voting.

679. I think you could do more to focus on the medical use in this survey. Arthritis is the biggest cause of disability in the US and also the easiest thing to treat with cannabis medicine, I thought it would have gotten a mention in the list of sign on conditions, rather than taking a back seat to ones that can't get you a legal

recommendation. Furthermore, I can't actually tell you how much cannabis flower or bud I'm using in a week because I use concentrates and it takes different amounts of flowers to procure the same amount of concentrate. Also, my consumption varies based on the effectiveness of the cannabinoid profile. I like a broad spectrum, personally, but I understand people are also big on isolating specific cannabinoids for their therapies. As far as recreational use goes, it looks like you've covered all the bases with lots of options for consumers to choose from. I just didn't think the questions really applied to me as a medical consumer, or rather, the options available as answers weren't applicable. I wasn't able to 'choose all that apply' on the question for 'cannabis use pattern.' I use 50-100mg doses up to three times a day, orally, as well as vaporized concentrates 3-5 times a day.

680. I think you should highlight the difference between and addiction and a dependency. I don't think marijuana is addictive in the classic sense, but I think it's effects and ease of use can cause people to become dependent on it for various situations, like using it as a long-term sleep aid and then struggling to sleep without it for a period.

681. I throw up when I'm stoned if I haven't smoked in weeks

682. I took medication for anxiety (mild/generalized) for several years. They worked well enough, but I always developed inability to orgasm, which was a deal breaker. Cannabis used prn has completely worked for me without any negative side-effects. In fact, I learned to enjoy exercise while using cannabis, lost 60 pounds and have remained a regular exerciser (without the need for cannabis). My use fluctuates depending on availability

and stress levels. Some weeks I use none, some I smoke up to 3 times a week.

683. I tried cannabis once at 19, but did not become a regular user until 24. I am glad that I let my brain fully develop before I started using regularly. I don't think people should habitually use until they are at least 21.

684. I understand I'm underage for smoking cannabis. In my opinion, it should be recreational and medical. Most effects have no va side. Alchohal is MUCH worse than cannabis, and cannabis is much more soothing.

685. I use cannabis all throughout the day. I do nearly all of my schoolwork and attend all of my classes high. It has no negative effect. My grades are the highest they have ever been.

686. I use cannabis because it enhances my enjoyment of other things, such as music, movies, books, etc.

687. I use cannabis exclusively for my pain related to a L5/S1 fusion that isn't so great.

688. I use cannabis for low back pain - topically and as alcohol (everclear) tinctures. Have only smoked it a few times in my lifetime. Also used it recreationally to relax with friends.

689. I use cannabis for medical reasons. Specifically to treat neuropathy pain & anxiety/depression.

690. I use cannabis recreationally because I enjoy the social/ creative benefits, but it also has helped to decrease anxiety that accompanies a long-term eating disorder.

691. I use cannabis recreationally because I enjoy the social/creative benefits, but it also has helped to decrease anxiety that accompanies a long-term eating disorder.

692. I use cannabis recreationally, but it's what makes me optimistic about my duties. With that said, I also believe that if someone smokes tobacco, it significantly affects their personal reactions to cannabis. (compared to someone who doesn't use tobacco) Specifically, I believe that cannabis induces anxiety to people who consume tobacco, but not those who don't. I don't believe cannabis has a negative effect on peoples' ability to think properly.

693. I use cannabis regularly while accomplishing my everyday tasks, with no noticeable I'll-effects

694. I use cannabis throughout the day. In the morning I need to stretch my leg, pylon fracture causes bone pain, and the arthritis makes it difficult to stretch my calf muscles. I have a consent unrest surrounding my childhood. And intermittent depression when I experience triggers. As I've learned how terpenoids work with our endocannabinoid system. I balance my intake as the day progresses. Morning I use a sativa and a CBD tincture to deal with the pain and stretch. After I treat my leg I finish exercise and eat. After breakfast I will medicate again with a sativa with a piney smell to start my day. This takes care of my anxiety and pain. I will use a small glass pipe throught the day to manage my pain and anxiety. In the evening I need to relax from the day and again deal with pain in my leg. I will medicate with a hybrid close to 50/50 with a citrus and earthy smell to go to bed and manage my pain. The biggest call I have to medicate is the pain experienced in my tibia and talus. An

issue I run into is I need to have CBD in my regiment to counter the psychoactive effects of THC. Without CBD or if I consume heavy indica plates lacking the terpenoids I need, I exacerbate my symptoms.

695. I use cannabis to ease the pain I have. I have never driven on cannabis and never will.

696. I use cannabis to increase my mood, relieve stress and relax.

697. I use it as a relaxer in the evening before bed, once all my 'chores' are done. In addition, it GREATLY helps reduce discomfort and stress when I am on my period.

698. I use it as a tool for creativity and to relieve tedium when coding. I got all my patents from using pot. Great for moving one's perspective allowing new ways of thinking about things. My code is much more succinct and works better with less bugs when I've programmed on pot. My music that I produce is also much better.

699. I use it because/when my boyfriend does.

700. I use it both alone and socially. With other users and around non users. Sometimes I get something out of the experience and other times I wish I hadn't smoked

701. I use it for anxiety and relaxation. I feel its so much better health wise than Xanax or valium.

702. I use it for my ms, and only use when going to bed, as it helps me sleep and helps my muscle spasms

703. I use it for Spiritual insight.. I understand that it helps break down habitual and social paradigms of thought. If I am spiritually in tune with myself I would likely have no need for an external drug. But because I find myself falling into limited beliefs due to my social and environmental surroundings I need to loosen by beliefs. I feel as though a different part of my brain CAN become active with appropriate intention. Also It appears to make a significant difference if the Cannabis has been grown in a spiritually healthy environment, as the 'vibes' the plant receives in it preparation effect the chemical structure.

704. I use it mainly to help me sleep. Conventional sleeping pills don't work well with me and don't help with the pain from my Rheumatoid Arthritis or Fibro. I do occasionally use it in a recreational manner but for the most part it allows me to stay off addictive opiate pain killers and keeps me working.

705. I use it to assist with insomnia and low appetite. It's also a fantastic social lubricant.

706. I use it to help me sleep at night and it helps with the pain of arthritis during the day. I'm a veteran with ptsd which cannabis helps with.

707. I use it to help relax after a long day at work with no ill affects in the morning. Sleep great!

708. I use mariguana for chronic pain

709. I use Marijuana because i like the effect. I feel that it cleans me out and i enjoy my own world in private with nature and natural surroundings. I can become a lot more sensitive as Marijuana

increases my awareness. I think that Marijuana should be available in abundance and that society has totally misjudged its usefulness and that people should be free to use it .

710. I use more often when I'm alone than with other people. I enjoy Cannabis when I get home from work or school if I know I don't have to go out again. I enjoy Cannabis before watching movies or TV, but not before reading. I enjoy cleaning and music more while using Cannabis, my sex drive improves, my anxiety level decreases (I'm a full time student with a part time job). I'm creative, I think critically, I appreciate nature and beauty more when I use Cannabis.

711. I use only CBD tinctures or capsules with little or no active THC. I don't 'get stoned' from these products, nor would I wish to. Prior experience has shown that I react very poorly to THC (increased anxiety/paranoia, inability to focus or function normally in any capacity).

712. I use to have seizures. I use to have insomnia. I use to have bouts of depression. Not any more thanks to marijuana.

713. I used cannabis in my senior year of high school for recreational use only, but i quit when i graduated. But when i went to xxxxxxxxxxxxxxxxx i played a lot of basketball and twisted my foot real bad. I hopped on one foot back to my dorm, elevated it and put ice on it and took aspirin. It didn't help much, most of the pain was still there. Two hours later a friend of mine stopped by because he herd what happened. He gave me an indica joint and said this should work. I smoked it and with in 5 min my pain level went from 8.5 to 1.5. This happened in 1989, and my friend laughed at me when i said ' The government

can't keep a lid on this forever, in some form or another this will be legal'. I never new cannabis had such medical potential.

714. I used cannabis to get off 19 different prescription medications. Eating it has helped me to 'accidently' get healthier. When I eat it, I need to inhale much less and I feel healing. I still inhale it for pain and anxiety control as needed. But when I have the supply to eat, I no longer need to inhale it nearly as much. I believe I have difficulty stopping it, because the surgeries that left me in a debilitated condition require medication until I am fully healed, rather than an addiction to the medication. I have an endocannabiniod system that has been severely damaged and requires supplementing.

715. I used it mostly recreationally, until I got sick, now most use is medical.

716. I used it vaporized during pregnancy for EXTREME nausea (I would have been hospitalized for manutrition), to GREAT effect. I could not keep down any food without it, it helped me be able to eat good meals and grow healthy children, instead of wasting away and risking my childrens health. I see no effect on my children, and lately have little desire to consume it regularly, but enjoy an occasional puff with friends.

717. I used marijuana a few times in high school/college, and didn't touch it again until two years ago. I now use it occasionally. As a former tobacco user that abused alcohol in my mid-20's, I know I have a high propensity for substance abuse. Marijuana is the one mind-altering substance I have not experienced any withdrawal symptoms from, and that I'm able to use 'normally.' My normal use patterns are to use it on occasional weekends

(about every other week), and on an occasional weekday if I'm having difficulty sleeping. My usual reasons for use are to relax and relieve stress, and to enhance sexual pleasure.

718. I used pot for fun during highschool. I loved it. Now I use just a tiny bit at night to unwind and have a deeper sleep. I get paralyzing anxiety if I smoke during the day and try to have normal interactions with people. I simply cannot do this anymore. I am not addicted and never have had a problem with not smoking. I usually prefer not to. It does help cope with things and does help my mood and PMS. I do not believe it is addicting, however- my boyfriend is addicted to it. This is due to addiction to substance. He used it to get off of heroin and now he just 'needs something' to fill in the missing gaps when things aren't going well. He does however experience withdrawal symptoms and I can tell you the main one is serious anger (he has serious anger issues since childhood anyways) but the agitation associated with withdrawal is far worse. Marijuana has actually saved my life (not literally) when I had a severe severe severe ear infection that rendered me incapable of walking. I was under sever vertigo and nausea and not even several doses of Dramamine worked. Marijuana did wonders. Good tip for vertigo/nausea sufferers!!!!

719. I used to be very fearful of Cannabis until I did ample research, which encouraged me to try it. When I tried it, I realized that it was even better than expected. It is very euphoric after a hard, stressful day. Depending on the strain, I felt very creative and I came up with very insightful ideas while high. Another thing I would like to mention is that it allows deep introversion. I feel like I can analyze my life and how to improve it while I am high. It allows me to focus very deeply on one task or thing, but focusing on multiple things is difficult.

720. I used to exclusively use cannabis as a Rasta sympathetic person and as a partner to a militant Rasta. During that time, I smoked every day, partly as a spiritual practice and partly as a habit. I did not drink alcohol during that time, which lasted about 5 years. After my mother saw me high and I felt ashamed, I quit completely and didn't smoke for a few years. Now, I do it occasionally, but I have to really be in the mood. I find that smoking cannabis makes me more conscious of my inner self, so when I'm not in the mood for being that aware of my inner self, I end up feeling self-conscious and paranoid.

721. I used to like it more when I used while also taking Zoloft. I don't know if my enjoyment was linked to that or if it is strain-dependent.

722. I used to smoke a lot more than I do now - every day. I can't afford to do that anymore. I never had a problem stopping and I've discontinued usage several times for 6 mos to a year without an issue. I can stop smoking cannabis, but not tobacco. It does make me more creative, and I miss that but after awhile, I find my own creativity, again. I do not like alcohol. I prefer cannabis over alcohol. No hangover and no aches and pains in my joints these days - in fact those feel better. I have always been able to function just fine after smoking. I think it affects different people in different ways though - depending on one's body chemistry. Thanks!

723. I used to smoke cannabis multiple times a day everyday, but in recent months my use has gone down to slightly less than once a day on average. Before bed to help with sleep.

724. I used to smoke cigarettes, while stopping I started smoking

more weed to compensate, but now I am slowly starting to slow down on consumption. I start vaporizing a lot more now, but I still selected bong because it is really the way I used to smoke the most with. What is great with vaporiser is that you can use the vaped weed to make edibles afterwards so its like recycling.

725. I used to use over the counter pain pills for menstrual cramps and PMS symptoms and especially to help me sleep. It quiets my racing thoughts before bed and I sleep a full night. So after a stressful day sometimes I feel like I need to take a small smoke as I get home to help me wind down and relax. I also have self-diagnosed disordered eating and I go through episodic occurrences of exercise/calorie fixation, diet control, and no appetite. When I smoke cannabis during those times I 'snap out of it' and reevaluate my negative self talk and see more realistically my body weight and self-image. Those episodes occur up to 3 times per year lasting around 3-5 weeks at a time. Cannabis helps me to feel hungry and interested in enjoying food and motivates me to think about taking care of my body and soul. During that time I will use more frequently to help recover so I can try to keep up a normal life (aka sleep better and participate in social activities instead of turning them down to save calories and exercise more)

726. I usually binge smoke for a week or so and then quit for a while, so my frequency of use statistics may be somewhat different from others.

727. I usually do not dream, but when I sleep soon after smoking I dream more frequently. Light pre-sleep use vastly increasing my feeling of restfulness upon waking up.

728. I usually only smoke at night or when I get home from work and i use it to destress, clear my head but also to deal with depression and i swear it helps me with my acid reflux and indigestion/heartburn.

729. I very rarely use cannabis, use it to de-stress every month or two, I would use it more but I feel it effects my thinking which I don't like

730. I wake up with nausea if I do not smoke cannabis within an hour of waking it increasingly gets worse. I'll smoke about .1-.15 gram and the nausea disappears within 10 minutes. If I have a migraine I will smoke about .05-.1 and lay down/ relax and the migraine will go away within 30-45 mins. Although I smoke for medical use/relief, I do smoke at a recreational level too.

731. I want it to be legalized so that I will no longer be seen as a ctiminal in the eyes of the law. Cannabis will always be a part of my life.

732. I want this marjuana or cannabis use to be taken out from society. This is killing people and destroying younger generation. Do you think a cannabis user will be hired by a cooperate office of a reputed firm. Every individual need to pass drug test. There are lot of ways to make money. Not by selling drugs.

733. I want you to know that I smoke weed only when offered. I have no addiction or need for weed. Depending on the setting ..affects reactions of the drug (around good people,at a concert ,outside at night,outside day time , music,no music,etc also, hallucinations sometimes depends on setting. When I get

really upset and I'm fighting with my bf I will walk away and smoke weed to calm down. It increases my thinking and makes me want to make everything better and work on communication. I all of a sudden see the world on a lighter note. Everything is better it almost feels like. I am a musician ..I can write music a MIlLLION times better after smoking a joint. My brain gets very creative and makes me want to work on singing and playing.

734. I wanted to relieve the muscle pain from the injury without use of prescription drugs. But I find it is hard to sort through info on internet about different strains. Yet some look like they would be helpful esp for bone growth - but what strain, what dosage, what side effects? I hope you can offer more specific info for the non recreational user. I have been relying on info from retailer.

735. I was a recreational user in the beginning. As an adult I started to realize other benefits from cannabis besides getting high. It helped with my day to day pain and stress. After an incident in the military it helped me deal with PTSD. I used it throughout the time I was in the military. I was even court-martialed for it. Since being diagnosed with heart issues I have found it to be the one thing that does not interfere with my heart meds. I use it now to help me sleep, not have nightmares, and to relax. It helps me manage being in pain and anxiety 24/7. It helps me to keep my nutrition level up and meds down. Otherwise I would be sick to my stomach all the time. For me personally I think it's the best medication available. I would rather use cannabis than take pharmaceutical prescription meds. I have seen cannabis help others as well. I believe that it should be legal throughout the country. PTSD patients specially veteran's

should all have access to cannabis. I am a strong supporter of cannabis legalization and use.

736. I was a test subject as a young child for adhd drugs (mainly being amphetamines) that actually made things worse. I substituted with cannabis and even my parents noticed a positive difference(they used to be very against its use until then). Hope this helps. :-)

737. I was a troubled kid growing up. I tried to commit suicide on more than one occasion. I could not handle society. When I got older, I decided to smoke marijuana one day after I had given up on everything. That moment saved my life. I had never experienced a level of clarity like that before. To this day I self-medicate with it because it helps me in so many ways. I have suffered seretonin syndrome and privately discussed with my doctor that I smoke marijuana. They saw no problem with the situation and considered it a good alternative. I am currently unemployed due to a random life circumstance - otherwise I'd be working full time.

738. I was born with a connective tissue disorder that was not diagnosed for 47 years. I started smoking cannabis at a very young age. It made me feel better when I was ignored by doctors and received no help. I think I would be in horrible shape by now without it.

739. I was born with a host of anxiety disorders, i had a very hard school life until i started using cannabis which allowed me to better understand peoples emotional states and allowed me too slow and focus on tasks which i'd otherwise be distracted from or too stressed to undertake. It also ended my long battle with

an OCD tick where i had to touch things multiple times or risk a paralysing illogical fear. This tick returns when i stop using cannabis for a period of 1-2 weeks.

740. I was diagnosed with fibromyalgia after surgeries, epidural injections in c-spine (along with a nerve ablation). I went to PT several different times, sometimes for up to 6 months. Post knee-surgery and several injections, my knee was worse. I finally received a 'gel' injections which helped much. They wanted me to have an injection into a hip with a radiologist. My 2nd opinion otho surgeon said I 'qualified' for hip replacement, even though they didn't recommend it.

741. I was diagnosed with panic disorder in 1997, years before I started using marijuana. Years later, I was able to get off of my anti-depressant by substituting marijuana. I also used marijuana to treat morning sickness during 3 pregnancies.

742. I was diagnosed with RA 8 years ago and was prescribed MMJ by my ND 2 years ago for pain. Since then I have been off all prescription meds and have been pain free most of the time. Before arthritis I was a avid runner, but had to stop because of the pain.Since starting MMJ therapy I have resumed running and Im now currently in the best shape of my life. MMJ has been a miracle for my RA and has improved many other areas in my life as well. Many positive side effects!

743. I was given less than a year to live in 2008. I started using high doses of cannabis for symptom relief. It allowed me to get off 27 pills a day and no longer need a wheelchair.

744. I was in recovery for 17 years when my medicine started

making my hair fallout - I started researching and talking to people about the benefits of cannabis. I had always been an advocate but was also ingrained that I couldn't and shouldn't do any drugs. I researched and researched and talked and talked. I tried to go off all my anxiety and depression meds but cannot yet. Cannabis helps me not need klonopin as much and it makes me happy BUT I cannot go off my last med - not until I have options to different strains of cannabis. Right now I am stuck with whatever I can find.

745. I was on 10 psychotropic drugs by the time i was 19. When i found cannabis, i ended all of those forever. My quality of life has been greatly improved because of cannabis. It is also good for the soul. In self reflection on how to be a better me and in relationship with other, nature and unity.

746. I was on bipolar pharmaceutical medications costing $2000/ month for about 10 years (ending in 2004). My quality of life is much better since I began using Cannabis for the headaches, migraines, insomnia, pain, and lack of appetite.

747. I was prescribed marijuana for a chronic pain condition caused by a birth defect. I am unable to drink alcohol and I hate taking opioids and muscle relaxers all the time.

748. I was prescribed Stratera in the 5th grade. This caused me too lose 45 pounds over a few months. When I reached high school I always complained about my inability to enjoy food and supply my body with proper nutrition. A close friend recommended I try cannabis to alleviate the problems I was having due to the medicine. Since then I have regularly combated the ill effects due to the various medicines and pills with cannabis.

749. I was raised by my grandparents, strict republicans, during the Reagan Administration. I fully participated in the Just say No club, and was raised to fear this plant. I chose to go against everything I was ever taught, after a failed 9 Month treatment regiment for Hep C that has left me without a ability to live a normal life. The meds they offered me were Methadone, and Oxycontin. I did not see those as a viable option as I had three daughters who were teenagers, I weighed under a hundred pounds, and was born premature, addicted to heroin, and had to spend over 45 days in the ICU as an infant going through withdraw. The addicted mind does not forget, and I was not willing to risk it. So I chose cannabis. I started going to the dispensaries, but was not comfortable with their lack of knowledge, testing verification for pathogens was lacking, and since my immune system is compromised I could not risk that so my caregiver began growing for me. I now only use what is grown for me. Every aspect of the plant life, from seed to end product results, are detailed, documented. The soil is custom blended, the microbes that are used are from a reliable source, the water is ph balanced, Every aspect of the grow is VITAL and not understood. Every plant used is chosen for a specific reason, terpenes, ratios of CBD to thc, My usage depends on the day, weather, sleep paterns, fatigue waves, but I consume daily, If I miss or just dont consume for whatever reason my body will slowly shut down, hands will cramp in, back muscles cramp up, ankles and feet ache and hurt to the point of inability to walk or put pressure on them without severe pain. The most I have weighed in 10 years is 118 and that was while I was on steroids for a severe rash over a third of my back from sun exposure that lasted 3 weeks. Most people do not know I even consume, even those who have known me for a couple of years. I do not get the red eyes, the stoned swollen eyes,

the munchies, cottonmouth (VERY RARELY), paranoid, or any negative side effect honestly. This is truly my medicine, I use it like a dietary supplement. I average about 500mg of THC/CBD a day through edibles, and between 4-10 1/8 gram bowls/joints a day of a 14%CBD to 6 %THC Flowers, with 3 grams of oil at 2Omg CBD per Gram. I believe in the full plant spectrum, where terpenes, and a balance of all cannabinoids not just THC/CBD and fatty acids (coconut oil gram capsules) all play an intricate part in the healing properties of the plant.

750. I was raised in rural tx & alcohol is everywhere and had done terrible things to people I love. My world flipped when I discovered this amazing plant that saved not only my life but my mothers after we both went through colon/bowel problems. For me all pharmas are gone and have been in remission for 5 years, my mother has cut her meds in half and is in great shape even after removal of her colon. We dont live in a mmj state and live in fear of crimes for something so beneficial.

751. I was really depressed before I tried cannabis for the first time there isn't really any reason for it . I started smoking and had a whole new outlook on life which is still happening after 11 years of daily smoking if it wasn't for weed I would probably be an alcoholic and hate life but instead I'm happy and lead a pretty proproductiveductive life. I think if everyone would smoke there would be a lot less jerks in the world. Also I'm using my tablet to do this survey so the slider bars will not slide. But all my symptoms are almost completely better with cannabis. I'm against pills so I'm so happy there is such a beautiful thing as cannabis or life would suck.

752. I went through the Doctor's regimen of things that I should do.

We found out that I'm allergic to the fillers in pills. I just got sicker & sicker...I first started w/coconut infused w/marijuana suppositories so I would quit throwing up. Once that happened I started smoking 1 gram/night to sleep. I was introduced to tincture, but didn't like the smell or taste, so we learned how to make hard candy using the tincture as the medicine. It has worked really well for several years & now I deal w/pediatric hospice patients. I'm very grateful for those who went before me and learned all of these interesting facts so that I had a base to go off of.

753. I work for xxxxxxxxxxxxxxxxxxxxxxxxxxx I am a recreational user up to my ears in the MMJ industry and I love my work because of the sense of purpose I now have.

754. I work in substance abuse treatment and mental health. No one comes in just for marijuana addiction. Marijuana just keeps people afloat while they can't do their harder drug of choice. It's danger is that they are usually not successful at stopping their harder drug of choice if they don't stop marijuana.

755. I would be asking specifically about side effects of cannabis use. the positive and the negative. what people what, what they avoid. you need questions about how people get their cannabis and what would serve them better questions ask if people realize that side effects are somewhat strain dependent and do they have adequate choices in their buying experience. a question numerically asking them how many strains are available to them in a week say. I have a med card in cali and mi but spend most of my time in a non med state and with only reliance on the black market I can't find adequate relief.

756. I would be taking a much higher amount of prescription drugs for my fibromyalgia without cannabis. I am grateful there is a medical marijuana program in my state. We will soon be getting dispensaries so I can start to experiment with different strains and see what works best for my condition.

757. I would highly encourage you to read/listen to these. Breaking Smart is the de-facto optimistic case for the future: http://breakingsmart.com/season-1/. Duncan Trussell is a loving, spiritual, psychedelic podcast that is truly amazing: http://duncantrussell.com/ If you seek to understand today you MUST understand the past, and this is the best, most incisive way to do that: www.dancarlin.com/hardcore-history-series/

758. I would prefer the legal medical option. I would prefer to try to topicals and have access to healthier routes of administration, as well as the ability to speak with a doctor who understands that not everyone wants to be an opiate addict and that this plant works. The first part of the questionnaire is confusing. I was not certain whether to answer from the perspective of 'life without cannabis' or 'life with it'. I tried to answer somewhere in the middle. When I do not have consistent access life is absolutely miserable because of the physical pain I live in, but I am not unhealthy outside of the chronic pain. Cannabis has been the only medication I have been able to take to for my back without experiencing severe withdrawal symptoms or having abnormal reactions to. Unfortunately it is not legal where I live and it is very difficult to find strains that actually help, but when you do you just wish you could grab the closest cop, doctor, or lawmaker and shout 'See this!? Before this I could not stand up without sharp shooting pains and neuralgia! And now look! I am walking and even longboarding

without a problem! Why is this wrong?' My sessions involve a few inhalations, not always holding in for five seconds. With nerve pain I have discovered that I get the most relief if I smoke a larger quantity before sleep. I wake up with minimal to no pain. If hypothetically a regular dosage is 0.3g per session then a 'large quantity' based on the increase I see to be effective in my case might be between 0.7-1g, Indica. High cbd sleepy strains to tend to work best for nerve and muscle spasms in my experience, especially at night for obvious reasons. Back pain has has reduced significantly with a combination of indica and sativa strains. The THC cannot be extremely high or both back pain and nerve pain increases for me. This is very difficult to have access to with consistency in a non-medical state, but I have replicated pain relief in this fashion many times over the years with the same results. The most negative part about cannabis is cost, legal risks, and social stigma all of which I hope to see change in the next five years.

759. i would probably use it more for my pain if it didn't interfere with my sleep and cause anxiety

760. I would rate my health 'excellent' if I did not have Atrial Fibrillation. First introduced 1957 (1 negligible hit), again in 1969, regular use since 1971. I use hemp regularly in small amounts, & find it relaxing, also enabling focus; I use it particularly when hiking & mountaineering.

761. I would say honestly that cannabis improves the quality of my life. Some of thes questions we're tough to answer because I didn't believe some of it applied to me. I do take cannabis because it helps me sleep, I'm a very worrysome person and it helps to calm me and I also have problems eating at times

which is a medical condition. I hope this helps, I was as honesty as possible

762. I wouldn't be able to eat without it. I have meds for anxiety and if I used them I'd be asleep 24/7. Pot doesn't do that to me. Its my savior!

763. I wouldn't consider myself a medical user. I dont NEED it for any condition. I like weed, it is fun, and makes me less of an asshole. My health has improved dramatically since I began to use cannabis. I have lost 30 pounds, mostly because I learned what true hunger was, I got more in touch with my body, and became far heatlhier as a result.

764. I'd love to see the results of this study!

765. I'd never smoked until my late 20's. Thought the whole medical thing might have some truth for cancer patients, but in general thought it was just hippies wanting to get high. After and accident ended up with years of nerve pain, after multiple surgeries and years of rehab eventually the doctors prescribed Lyrica. Although intended for seizures, it worked for my pain as well. The side effects were terrible though, and also meant we'd never be able to have kids. When searching online for various alternatives to Lyrica, cannabis was mentioned over and over. So tried it. Pain was totally gone, and the side effects were minimal relative to Lyrica.

766. I'm a fully-functioning professional in the xxxxxxxxxx industry, father who has helped raise two excellent teens (16 and 19 at present), committed volunteer currently a respected president of the board of our faith institution (where I know for

a fact that our executive director and our lead clergy member also get high). I am fortunate to live in xxxxxxxxxxxxxxxxx where recreational marijuana is legal, although - (a) I recently got a medical card b/c the rollout of legal recreational weed has been hampered here by supply chain issues and some poor decisions by government bodies, and (b) I still feel there is a stigma (but shrinking) over acknowledging weed usage. For example, I would offer many guest in my home a drink, but for very few would I offer a toke or an edible as an alternative.

767. I'm a mom & it really helps me with 2 kids under 5!!

768. I'm a mother of a 2 year old, though technically not employed

769. I'm a Navy Veteran and the use of cannabis has helped me tremendously with my PTSD and my anger issues. I've been smoking or consuming cannabis for almost everyday since 2006. I've never been healthier and happier. I eat a plant based diet and exercise, hike, do art and ride horses regularly. Cannabis has helped me deal with friends dying and life's incredible destructive hiccups. You asked if I thought cannabis is addicting, but never offered habit forming. There is a difference. I detoxed for two weeks and my moods where horrible and the lack of appetite and crazy vivid dreams is what finally got me to start smoking again. I had been convinced to 'give it up', guilted into thinking I was less of a person for relying on this 'plant'. Well it grows on this planet for a reason, and its for us to consume, and to help establish peace and understanding through out our planet and species.

770. I'm a parent of 2 children who I wouldn't be able to function through my health problems if it wasn't for cannabis. Yet I have to fear CPS due to this.

771. I'm currently using concentrates to maintain nerve pain from neuropathy and I am telling you no pharmaceuticals work better than cannabis to maintaining a normal life living with this type of disability.

772. I'm disabled & don't drive. I have neurological damage from chemo, allo transplant and associated drugs. I'm taking cannabis to control moderate to severe joint pain. I use 4 CBD Caps in 24 hrs. They are Harlequin: 6mg THC, 17mg CBD, 3mg other cannabinoids.

773. I'm forced to buy my marijuana on the street and all I can find is so expensive and POTENT. I'm not as ambitious being so 'stoned', I often opt to sit at computer rather than do the housework I regret not doing. I've various medical issues that would qualify me for medical herb, but I live in Wisconsin. My lifestyle and wardrobe suffers because I'm broke... I will buy weed before food (I weigh over 200 lbs)

774. i'm from new mexico. my licence is for pain.it works.i also have variable high blood preassure.it never goes up as i smoke.

775. I'm going to be here for hours! Firstly let me start of by saying that I believe cannabis should be decriminalised and taxation should be added and managed by the government (or local councils). This money should go to helping others with drugs issues and helping the society we live in as a whole (I know you guys are American too!) . As for myself, I'd say that cannabis is one of my main interests. It adds a level of depth and understanding that I believe nothing else matches. Regarding people that I know and spend time with, it seems to have some sort of effect on the way you think of life as a whole

and the universe (sure all stoners can agree that at one point or another we've sat there for ages talking about such random shit!) This definitely isn't in a negative way. Also one reason, especially in the UK, a lot of negative and not nice people seem to use cannabis for recreational use. This is one of the main reasons why cannabis doesn't really have the persona that it should. (these people I believe smoke it more than the other person has because they have the spare time, have easier access to the plant and are more likely to break the law.) Personally I tend to not smoke cannabis round people that don't like it or don't like the impact it has on me as a person. I don't have any issues with this. I have a xxxxxxxxxxxx brother who also smokes cannabis regularly and neither of us have had any mental issues. Also as I live in Britain, we do not have access to prescription cannabis over here as you probably know. As always when taking any mind/body alteration substances, it's always important to educate yourself with facts about it from various different sources and always take within moderation. I, and also others believe that others who take the substance believe that it can bring people together and allow them to interact as we like people that we can relate to. That's the way the human brain works! Hopefully one day we'll all be able to walk into our local coffee shop and buy a fat blunt and just sit with some friends and get high. Also legalizing/decriminalizing cannabis definitely could decrease crime rates, as alcohol consumers will make the switch permanently or just smoke it instead. Any other questions or updates ping me an email xxxxxxxxxxxxxxxxxxxxxxxxxxx. Fun little survey thanks. :)

776. I'm not in Washington state, I'm in PA

777. I'm not sure the 'immediate' effects question accurately represents the effects of cannabis overall, like the options would suggest. There should be a '1-2 hours after ingestion/ intake of cannabinoids' question for a better representation with many if not all of the same options, in my opinion. I do get the munchies, but not immediately after smoking. Also, what if I don't choose my flowers by any of those options? They are NOT medicine for me, but a substance much like alcohol or nicotine. For this reason, that question bothered me. I don't really care what I acquire, as long as it has THC in it.

778. I'm not sure what you need to know but here is some anecdotal information regarding my use. I consider myself a recreational user, but while I do mostly partake for fun or to relax, cannabis helps me a great deal in many different ways, the most important of which (to me) has been improved sleep. I have always struggled with insomnia which was primarily linked with stress. When I did sleep 50% of my dreams seemed to be nightmares and the majority of the other 50% were rarely happy and I often woke up feeling depressed or inadequate. Cannabis has helped me manage my stress, often by allowing me to see more creative or logical solutions, which has helped my sleep habits immensely. Likewise, as is largely known, cannabis suppresses how much I dream (while using daily I have maybe one or two dreams per week that I will vaguely remember the following morning) and because I am no longer having bad or unpleasant dreams, I often wake up feeling happy and hopeful with a much more positive and motivated outlook on life. Whether that is solely from no longer having bad dreams or from some other change in my life or a chemical change, I'm not quite sure. Cannabis has been a very positive force in my life. Since I started toking roughly one year ago I

have become more outgoing and made new and great friends due to our common interest (I'm very introverted and rarely make new friends), I have lost 30 lbs, I have been promoted at work, I went back to school (something I had been telling myself I would do for 4 years prior to using cannabis), and I have started managing my money better. Overall, I believe I have progressed more in various aspects of my life in the last year while using cannabis than in the previous 5 years combined. I can think of very little negative effects cannabis has had on my life. The only way I can say for certain that cannabis has affected me negatively is in regards to memory. It has in no way impaired me or disrupted my life, but I have always had a very good memory, whereas I now seem to regularly forget how long ago I did something, specific details regarding an event, or confusing events or details with other events or details.

779. i'm paralyzed on nearly 50% of my body cannabis is the only thing that helps eliminate spasticity and pain

780. I'm stoned

781. I'm transgender so assume the gender is true gender not AAB

782. I've been dealing with endometriosis for almost 10 years. I'm finally starting to get a handle on it. From the discovery of it with a horrible surgery and told I would never have children at the age of 26, it's been an uphill battle ever since. I have had approximately 8 different doctors over the years. All of them have prescribed me some form of narcotics. I've tried physical therapy, change of diet, exercise programs, running, yoga, Pilates, acupuncture, acupressure, massage therapy, hormone therapy, birth control pills, and MORE. It's been a battle. The

only, ONLY thing that has helped me in ANY way is smoking pot. I have more mental clarity, way less pain and stress from pain. I can drive my car and go to work, which I couldn't do while I was taking a Vicodin everyday. My body doesn't produce progesterone at all, so being estrogen dominant has put strain on personal relationships. But after smoking pot, I am a more balanced person. I don't get upset over small details. It's more of a live in the moment approach on life and everything is easier to deal with (for lack of better words). Depending upon where I am in my cycle, I can wake up in the morning and not be able to move. My lower back hurts so bad or the cramping is unbearable. I have to reach for the heating pad and lay there for another 20 mins before I can actually move. Once out of bed, I'll take one to two hits and within minutes the edge of the pain is gone. The mental stress of the pain is gone. My muscles can relax and so can my brain. I may have to take some Aleve or ibuprofen to help, but it's not Vicodin, Percocet or Tramodol which is what I used to take every single day for over 5 years. So yes, do I also use it recreationally? But it's truly because without it I literally wouldn't be able to get out of bed some days. I wouldn't be able to carry on a conversation without crying or yelling for no reason because my hormones are all out of whack and I don't have mental control. I am a huge fan. I've always been a recreational smoker but in the last almost three years, I've truly discovered what this plant can do for me. To me, it's a miracle. I hope this information helps. As much as it has helped me. Thank you for your work in this field and trying to make it more accessible. xx from xx

783. I've been in two car accidents while under the influence of marijuana, the second time with 32 grams of high grade cannabis in the car, and the other person received the ticket

both times and I've never been arrested for anything. I was extremely stoned for the accident where I had some in my car but I must not have looked like it. I was the one to call the police, for both accidents, and within five minutes 3 state trooper vehicles pulled up with two cops in each car. But they never asked to look in my vehicle. Also, alcohol is far more dangerous. I've had numerous friends, relatives, classmates, and co-workers that have died from the direct or indirect effects of alcohol. Also, many more have been imprisoned from alcohol use. But to this day I haven't had anyone I know die from the direct or indirect effects of marijuana. And have only known a few to go to jail or be on probation from cannabis. I don't think I've ever even heard of anyone that has died from the direct effects of using marijuana, either.

784. I've been prescribed xanax for anxiety, have opted to stop taking it for cannabis which I think is psychologically addictive, but still less so and less damaging than taking xanax any time anxiety arises or to sleep. Overall I think that it improves outlook on life and can have a positive motivating effect if controlled, like anything.

785. I've been smoking cannabis for 40+ years, both medically & before that, recreationally. I retired from a government xxxxxxxxxxx job after 35+ years & never felt that I couldn't function at least as well as my non-using peers.

786. I've been smoking off and on since I was 14, in 1974. I actually have never had issues related to smoking pot, never been arrested for it, never had it interfere with my work, parenting, marriage, relationships. As I mentioned above, smoking totally alleviated my hot flashes and other menopausal discomfort. No

side effects. I am now post menopausal and feel fine.

787. I've been using sleeping pills for almost 25 years every night and can't sleep without them. Started substituting indicas (combo edible and vape) and it's working.

788. I've given the information i feel is pertinent. some questions, while i am sure have meaning for you, don't work for me, and i'm not submitting that information here. thanks for working on this. this is truly a wonderous plant & it's medicinal uses could benefit many. p.s. i do not claim to use this medically. i do believe i would qualify for anxiety issues alone. not to mention ruptured discs & ibs. i've great personal experience with cannabis & like many others highly recommend the use for many aches, pains & simply to relax.

789. I've had asthma since I was young, and even when new to cannabis, noticed how much easier it was to breathe after smoking. It felt like I had just had an albuterol breathing treatment. As I got older and did more research, I came to understand that this was due to the bronchodilatory and expectorant effects caused by some of the alkaloids in cannabis.

790. I've had issues of rug addiction other than cannabis: cocaine and opiates

791. I've never liked being stoned, and just recently began using medical marijuana upon the advice of a friend. I've found that Indicas work amazingly well for the pain associated with my spinal stenosis and spinal cord compression, as well as for insomnia (as long as I ingest the indica rather than smoking it) and for the post-traumatic anxiety I've suffered for years. And

with indica's I don't feel high, just calm. I haven't even tried sativa, as I've been told that it generally has the effects I used to associate with marijuana, such as paranoia and the feeling of being stoned.

792. I've smoked pot on a regular basis for 40 years. I have an excellent job, a nice home and three college educated children.

793. I've sold weed in cities where it hasn't been decriminalized. I had clients who were your average stoners, and I've had clients who used it medicinally. I was very close to the clients who used it medicinally, and i can tell you that they weren't themselves when they weren't high. Two of them in particular were unable to function if they went long periods without weed (not attending class, not doing homework, not physically active, stayed inside all day being miserable).

794. I've substituted alcohol when cannabis is not available. It doesn't really help. Cannabis use makes me aware of physical tension that I ignore or block out when I am not using it.

795. I've suffered from anxiety, depression and suicidal and self harming practices since I was a young teen. I never used drugs or tobacco products, or drank until well after I was an adult. I waited to smoke cannabis until it was voted on in Washington state and became legal to smoke. I have been smoking for three months and have seen a tenfold improvement in my anxiety and depression management. I have also used it to treat myself after a whiplash diagnosis. My whiplash has cleared up and I was able to completely discontinue the use of prescription painkillers and muscle relaxers early on.

796. I've survived xxxxxxxxxxxxxxx cancer, HEP C, 3 heart attacks. Wife of 32 years divorced me right after harsh xxxxxxxxxxxxxxx cancer treatments. Could not swallow liquids for 3.5 yrs, solid food 5.5 yrs. Fried from chemo I have cognitive disorder (no short term memory, lack of focus & concentration and more...) and have been considered permanently disabled since 1998. I have had several stress related heart attacks and one minor stroke. I am almost blind in my left eye and am developing glaucoma. I am a choke hazard and must have an aide to make it thru each day safely. I can't ven remember to eat & take my pills. I am very forgetful and get lost easily. I am unable to safely drive a car any longer. I suffer from severe vertigo, arthritis, fibromyalga and more.... I even attempted suicide in late xxxxx. Cancer sucks and has destroyed every aspect of my life. If it were not for my illegal consumption I would not be alive today!

797. I've witness marijuana help others as well as myself with ADHD, PTSD,HIV and Cancer.

798. Iam on medical pot and I see no reason that weed is illegal because it's good for me but bad for others even if we smoked off the same plant!!! What the fuck just make weed legal and stop all the bullshit

799. If any addiction is due to boredom. When I was younger I would masturbate to pass the time, now if I have nothing to do I smoke. I try not to smoke for that reason. I usually try to have a very productive day or week and then light it up as a reward for being so damn awesome. I am a pretty good mathematician. When I smoke I end up either doing some excersice or proving some theorems on my whiteboard. Man, I am happy.

800. If it was not for Cannabis I would be on pills for depression, anxiety as well as an eating disorder. Cannabis brings me back to a happier place which the pills do but with the side effects as well as the other crap that comes with it.

801. If people were educated about marijuana and the affects then people will not fear the drug. Also the age for cannabis use should be around 25 years old because eye development stops around that age. Educated population = better population as a whole. The propaganda needs to stop and people need to realize that it will not make people gay or kill children.

802. If used appropriately it can be very helpful to certain people as long as it is not abused.

803. If you educate people on responsible use there is potential for many benefits to society as a whole - people generally tend to overindulge for no reason and thus get all the negative side effects you have listed in your survey, its not a drug that needs to be abused to be effective and people don't get that.

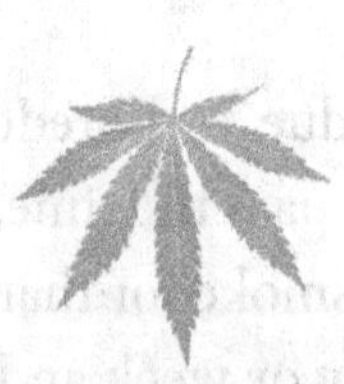

804. Im a activist for legalisation...my twitter account is xxxxxxxx and i regularly share articles, statistics and studies from around the world relating to all issues of cannabis.

805. Im a very light user, only once at bedtime, I take a few puffs to relax, help with my pain and allow me to sleep. Pot is the best medicine ever for stomach problems, pain, and to help with mood. It should have been legal all these years!! Its only a natural growing weed. I dont think the government should have the power to stop people from smoking weeds if they want to. God put Pot here for us to have. Who are we to argue with Gods creation!!!

806. Immediate effects are not a problem and are a great stress reliever, and can even make me more articulate, energetic, creative and social. The primary downside for me a lack of motivation, decrease in communication skills and lack of desire to socialize the *following day* after use. These effects generally last up to a day and a half after use, and quickly diminish after abstinence. After about 5 days of abstinence, I am usually back to 100%.

807. improves my over all outlook on life, improves on my anxiety. more sociable

808. Improves my quality of life

809. In all of recorded history, cannabis use has not caused a single death...ever.

810. In college, pot mostly made me want to sleep. I did not smoke for many years as I raised my family. A few years ago, I was

having issues with sleep/pain, and I started using edibles. It is wonderful to get a full nights sleep, and the cannabis also helps with my arthritis pain.

811. In countries and states without medical access induces many of the negative symptoms related to Cannabis such as Paranoia, once again a result of prohibition. I began using Cannabis originally due to extremely depressing circumstances in my life. Ever since I've used it to improve my quality of life through reducing stress and increasing motivation for exercise and general positivity including sleeping for longer hours than previously (7-10 Hrs). I feel unaccepted by local society and wonder if I am ever going to be able to receive safe access to medical standard quality Cannabis rather than funding and growing organised crime for poorly produced product. It's a shame that young individuals like myself are forced to risk my potential future career just to receive a substance that substantially improves the quality of my life, only adding to the circle of continuous depression that riddles the lives of many in areas of prohibition.

812. In general, more gender options for surveys, please.

813. In my experience using Cannabis I have become wiser and more aware of what should warrant medicinal use, not all varieties of the herb have helped me in certain downfalls, some mixes of the active compounds CBD & THC have polar effects to other hybrids. I can only learn and apply my knowledge to what truth I know, the fact is that over 90% of the bud on the streets could be this or could be that, Trainwreck for example comes in many forms such as a 50/50 I/S hybrid, 40/60 S/I hybrid, 90/10 indica dominant hybrid etc. Real medicinal use of Cannabis can only

come from trial & error or from a reputable source, the fact is the streets are not a reputable source, dispensaries ARE! KNOW WHAT YOUR TAKING, KNOW WHERE IT CAME FROM, KNOW WHY YOU TAKE IT AND BELIEVE IN THE TRUTH THAT IT HELPS PEOPLE!

814. In my experience, recreational Cannabis use in NOT for everyone! I have seen individuals unable to drive, falling asleep, hallucinating, acting strangely like they're lost in another dimension, etc. One should definitely be aware of his reasons for using Cannabis and whether or not the effects are mostly positive.

815. In my personal use I think Cannabis is an excellent substance. Quality of life improves for myself and pain is more manageable than using just over the counter Ibuprofen. Normally I would be taking 800 - 1200 Mg of Ibuprofen for Arthritis and other joint pain, but I can use much less in the way of Cannabis (1g - 3g) per 'Session' and be able to function in a better manner. I would rather smoke Cannabis to manage all my sports injuries from the past, then to use ~1000mg of Ibuprofen of other NSAID to treat my pains. I still use Ibuprofen, but at a much reduced rate to 400 - 800mg of ibuprofen maybe 2 times a week.

816. In my youth (15-25yrs old) my use was for different purposes. As I have gotten older, I understand the medicinal aspect much better, and that I was self medicating before. My quality of life is improved now that I am not nauseous all the time, I can keep my food down, and I have far more energy to do activities. Legal or not, I would continue to use marijuana as part of my medical regime.

817. In one of your questions you asked about driving...I don't drive... In other question you asked about addiction. ..I don't think there addicting to the point of nicotine, but I notice if I don't smoke it affects my moods....thank you for putting this survey out there

818. In one question I said that Cannabis is addicting and in another I said I did not know. I do not think it is as addictive physiologically/psychologically as it is socially and habitually.

819. In regard to the box 'Highest level of education completed', I've only _completed_ high school. But I think it is important to note I'm currently in my last year to complete an Associate and Bachelor degree with plans to pursue graduate studies.

820. IN regards to addiction treatment - I was FORCED to go as a result of a plea deal for an arrest relating to drug possession - when asking about drug treatment you should clarify if it is a personal decision or a required course of action from a court system. IN relation to addiction - one can be dependent on a drug without being addicted. My body prefers to have cannabis (IMO it requires the substance to be whole) so when I am without it the irritability loss of appetite and nausea i feel is my body acclimating to the loss of the compounds found in cannabis

821. In regards to the cardiovascular symptoms that many people say cannabis gives; the feeling is about the same as being sexually aroused.

822. in the 60' 70's it was all about recreation - now it is for health, sleep and pain reduction

823. In the category for short term affects I want to clarify and point out that some of my answers may sound contradictory, for example when I stated that sometimes when I take cannabis I feel motivated and want to stretch and other times I feel tired and want to relax. I chose both option due to the various affects cannabis has. The THC and CBD levels have a lot to do with the mood that is created. Environment and other personalities can affect the type of 'high' I get. Thanks for doing this survey!

824. In the past, I self-medicated with cannabis to help with low thyroid and and anemia symptoms. Smoking would give me an energy boost so that I could clean my house and cook for my family. I'm sure there are many women like me, who go undiagnosed or undermedicated for their hypothyroidism because of doctors dogmatic reliance on the TSH test. I've found that Bastyr doctors are no better at this than conventional doctors. Now that I have adequate thyroid hormones, I don't have to rely on cannabis for energy.

825. In the survey you ask if, in our opinion Cannabis is addictive. I answered, no. But honestly I think that anything can be addictive and abused. Even if Cannabis isn't habit forming or has little to no withdrawal effects.

826. Include wooden pipes in survey. I get a lot of yard work done.

827. Ingesting an edible before bed has helped my sleep more than any other thing or supplement. It's been a life saver. Smoking or vaporizing helps with stress. I grow my own organically and make my own edibles.

828. Initiative 502 states that when the law was passed, medicinal

marijuana patients wouldnt be affected by it and any laws that were made with it, further more this would be a much better survey if it had a few more options for the majority of it. thank you

829. Instead of lumping all cannabis together you should be more specific about type (sativa/indica or sativa/indica dominant hybrid) for each question. You only had one question on the survey about that. I can get anxious when smoking sativa or sativa dominant cannabis, but I avoid those strains. Medical dispensaries and growing scholarship around strains has made it far easier for me to choose a strain that works for me. Also if I give you my ethnicity, gender, zip code, initials, my mother's maiden initial, the 1st letter of my birth city, and the last two digits of my birth year, my marital status, income, drinking habits and social proclivities I would imagine you would be able to find out who I was. Not that you are looking, but information on the internet is like pee in a pool, you can't really get it out. So, I gave a fake one that I can remember if I ever participate in another study. I dunno, maybe I am just paranoid from all the weed I've been smoking.

830. It ain't so bad.

831. It allows me to relax.

832. It can coincide with normal life. And is non dependent i have stopped three times for over a year stretches with no qualms.

833. it can have different effects. like if i'm feeling lazy and take a puff i might get motivated. if i'm very motivated and i take a puff it might make me distracted. if i smoke before i sleep i cannot

remember my dreams. i stop for 30 days a couple times a year and when i do my dreams become more vivid and i remember them. i will often not smoke for the vivid dreams.

834. it clears my head after a long day and helps me relax and not take the world so serious. it helps bring out my silly creative side everyone loves. it helps so much with stress, who doesnt have stress?

835. It cures cancer

836. It doesn't help directly a whole lot with pain but it's been very helpful to reduce stress, improve relaxation and calm (including ability to sleep) -- which are constant side effects of having multiple painful chronic illnesses. I'm very thankful it's now more easily accessed and purchased - in various forms (I prefer not to smoke).

837. it gives me what my prescription medications can't, relief

838. It has a very strong effect on back pain much better than the painkillers you can purchase

839. It has been my opinion that cannabis heightens one's emotions, similar to how it can heighten one's sense of smell). Like a psychedelic, the mental 'set' (as well as the physical 'setting', particularly if it's an obtrusive one!) of the user during a session should be considered when evaluating the mental effects of cannabis, particularly with regard to its use as a stand-in for antidepressants and anti-anxiety medications.

840. It has certainly made a positive impact on my daily life and the ability to do everyday things.

841. it has healed me and reduced chronic pain . the amount I use of non active thc herb will not be affordable if I have to buy it.

842. It has less side-effects than drugs I've had a prescription for and works better. The main problems with it are its legal status, price, and association with negative stereotypes. It needs to be widely accepted, as it is safer and more responsible than alcohol, tobacco and most prescription drugs.

843. It helps life become more vivid. I mean why can cigarettes and alcohol be legal that are well known for death and cannabis a form of nature grown from the earth be criminalized. The government is corrupt all they want is money and more casualties of drug overdoses and drunk people. As one I'm not for it, i see cannabis as a life saver a 'miracle herb'. All the money used to support cannabis would be used to create more jobs better revenue enhanced schools affordable colleges fixed roads and so on. I'm tired of hiding the world needs to wake up and realize it's not bad. If you don't like it then don't smoke it. Pretty much goes as if you were to smoke a cigarette. There is no contact high from second hand cannabis. I've been arrested for having a gram of cannabis. I'm not happy everyone's taxe dollars are going to a hard working man that gets arrested for no apparent reason it's ridiculous there's more things to worry about then cannabis like herion pills and drunk drivers. Wake up America!!

844. It helps live a better life

845. It helps me in many ways.

846. It helps me with pain and helps me not get addicted to pain medication

847. It helps pain and muscle spasms from a condition called Sydenham's chorea. It's quite an annoying disease

848. It is a better choice than alcohol and a more effective medicine than prescription drugs for my needs.

849. It is a foolish idea to legalise it's use in Canada and America. Cannabis is now full of GMO's and is created in glorified sunless labs. The plant is no longer sacred or respected as such. We should be using the whole plant and teach about its healing properties. Now the wealthy will use their monopolies and gain all the wealth cannabis is generating. The local drug dealer has lost his job!

850. It is a herb god created and it has less side affects than prescription drugs.

851. it is a miracle drug and has replace a handful of meds i once took. i can't sing it's praises enough

852. It is a no brainer, non toxic, no hangovers. Makes you chill, no drunken debauchery. If you have a problem with pot, then I have a problem with you!

853. It is far more beneficial than Alcohol, non addicting, and good to relax with

854. It is far safer and better for u than alcohol but is illegal think it's about time people deside there own choices rather than big corporation funded and run governments to be true 2 the people !!! Cancer is terrible disease we have a cure get it out there!!?!!

855. It is great as a stress relief. Muscle cramp relief. Stomach ache relief anti inflammatory snd more. Relaxing for me and helps me eat when I normally wouldnt want to.

856. It is ridiculous to allow alcohol to be legal when it has NO medical value, and keep Cannabis illegal when it has numerous capabilities. It's pretty sickening.

857. It is the healing of the heart and the creator of peace and unity.

858. It is the only thing that gives me an appetite.

859. It is useful as a replacement for many harmful meds wthout negative side effects and harm.

860. It is very difficult for me to come by. I tend to "feast or famine" so I can go months between having enough. I have found it to be a great mother's little helper as I am overwhelmed by my new life as a stay at home mom during the day and continuing to work outside the home evenings and weekends. I first used it in college to help with the pain of endometriosis. I immediately told my mom and doctor about this and they were supportive. I have continues to use it for pain, depression and to make my child's endless game of "you wear the hat" a bit more fun.

861. It is very important that organic medical grade marijuana remain available to the persons who need it for health and healing. I have used it successfully for 40 years for various health issues, including cancer. My mother used it for her glaucoma and her mother (who died at age 103) for her trigeminal neuralgia and other forms of pain. Both indica and sativa types have their specific uses. It is a very powerful healing herb in it's many

varying forms (tinctures, salves, oral, etc). I'm also a Bastyr patient and would appreciate Bastyr's support on the medical marijuana issue!

862. It is welcoming to see more legitimate scientific and educational focus on Cannabis in recent years - I hope and expect this trend will continue.

863. It keeps me calm and happy I need to smoke everyday I have been smoking pot for a long time I had bad times with drinking so I smoked pot instead...ive got athsma...It has weaned me off cocaine and keeps me off it...I need to smoke pot everyday

864. It needs legalized and taxed.

865. It needs to be legal.

866. It put my wife's seizure's into remission as well as a 14 year old boy I make oil for. The only thing evil about cannabis is... the people who made up the lies about it to bring on prohibition

867. It really helps with nausea and muscles cramps from the HVC. I was taking up to 5 Percocet a day for pain but now 1-2 a day when using cannabis. I get a burst of energy that allows me to function during the day. smoked it before it was legal here. so much better now. At least I know exactly what is and isn't in it.

868. It relaxes the body while stimulating the mind.

869. it seems a safer bet than Risperdal and Seroquel and binds on the same receptors. Since these prescriptions cause movement disorders with improper withdrawal, I strongly support the use

of cannabis. When it is indicated that people have a hard time stopping it's use, that is because of the receptors that it binds to. No one stops atypicals without disorientation or worse

870. it seems recreational cannabis stores has difficulty with suppliers and the cost would be triple. Why should the medical patients suffer?

871. It should be legal

872. It should be legal

873. It should be legal all around. Safer then alcohol.

874. It should be legal and it should be studied.

875. It should be legalised and available to all who feel the need to roll a spliff

876. It should not be a controlled substance. Use of cannabis can improve medical conditions in some people.

877. It should only be used in the privacy of your own home, not out in public. People in CA are allowed to grow FAR TOO MUCH for their own personal use which promotes illegal selling for monetary gain. There's no reason any single person needs to grow 50 plants (or even 10 for that matter) for personal use, that's ridiculous!

878. it simply meets all my needs both medically, and recreationally. im happy,fit, and well and thats all i really need i think.

879. it slows down my thinking and allows me to think more clearly and not over think a situation

880. It was a little hard to describe my experiences under the influence of cannabis because it varies for me each time I use it. For example, sometimes I am more social, sometimes less. Sometimes I am more active, sometimes more lazy.

881. It was difficult to know what boxes to check for 'short term effects' because even though many of the short term effects seem to contradict one another, a cannabis user could experience contradictory short-term effects when using different strains of marijuana. For example, one strain may make the user more social, when another could make the user less social. Some strains induce 'munchies', others do not, and so on.

882. it was hard for me to answer about choosing product from dispensary as I am my own grower/supplier for MANY years. In my eyes recreational is also medicinal use...stress kills its a fact, most rec users are trying to unwind or relax from perhaps a stressful day at work or raising kids...cannabis is this age's Valium...mothers little helper..the stigmata attached to cannabis use has kept many sick and the elderly from trying cannabis..prohibition must end...thank you for your time :)

883. It was hard to describe my 'short term effects' via the questionnaire considering each strain causes a completely different high. For those which give me more 'negative' side effects I usually do not purchase them again. So yes, I will experience negative side effects such as uneasiness, paranoia, etc, but rarely considering I know what I like. Also, I use cannabis as a pre emptive approach to anxiety and I have not

found it to be particularly helpful in say, a panic attack, but it's kept me from escalating to that point. On the opposite coin, it almost always eases feelings of depression.

884. It weirdly seems to keep me fitter/better looking? I've noticed that when I eat brownies I'm a lot less bloated looking and stay very lean. Although it does seem to be drying to the skin and possibly makes me look a little older.

885. It works great for menstrual cramps for women that have it more severe than others. Migraines as well just only for 30 min or so with very strong cannabis. It's just too much for so little amount what is the main problem for people that should be able to grow their own in apartments as well as homes.

886. it would be nice to know what strain i am buying instead of realing on what ever the dealers got :(some are better for my pain. i dont want to be a criminal but i cant handle the pain and over the counter pain relief irritates my stomach ulcers

887. It's a miracle plant and it is stupid the US government deems it a disgusting substance.

888. it's a plant that has numerous use's our government needs to stop the war on marijuana.

889. It's a profound shamanic spiritual tool, for people who choose to use it that way. One factor that was left out of your survey is coffee drinking. Coffee has an opposite spiritual effect of cannabis; coffee smokers typically smoke a lot more weed, and still don't achieve the same clarity of high. Also, people who have some experience with psychedelic drugs tend to understand how to use cannabis more efficiently. Thanks!

890. It's allright once in a while

891. It's an amazing plant with lots of positive benefits. When compared to the negative effects of alcohol, a legalized drug sold on street corners all across the world and advertised on TV, it's a laughable comparison.

892. It's an herb, like lavender or sage or oregano or whatever. It's a natural plant that should be grown as simply as people have herb gardens with basil, parsley, etc. I don't approve of the idea that the only way pot should be legal is through medical or commercial. It should be sold at farmers markets, not managed by the Bureau of Alcohol, Tobacco and Fire Arms. People shouldn't even profit on it. It's kind and gentle. Doctors, lawyers and PhDs smoke it. It's saved many a person from becoming an alcoholic, like in our parents' generations when pot wasn't around. People need to just let it grow and chill out. It's a prayer. It's spirit. It's better for your lungs than tobacco and cheaper now too. It could bring world peace. Just don't let the oligarchy and megacorps control it. That would suck.

893. It's fun

894. It's fun :)

895. It's great as long as you don't use it day in day out and take 2 week tolerance breaks every once in a while. It's all about not allowing your dopamine receptors to downregulate too much. Next to that I think everyone should use edibles or vaporizers, smoking it or using it with tobacco makes the drug so much worse than it actually can be, more damaging and also addictive, as your brain will anchor cannabis intake with nicotine intake,

which in my opinion could make you crave cannabis, while it's actually the nicotine that's being craved. Finally, I even think it has made me smarter in the long run, because I seem to be much more able to see things from other perspectives and see connections between things ever since using cannabis recreationally for about 1-2 times a week (with regular breaks).

896. It's great for some people, it's not addictive and it's a great attribute for people who are ill.

897. It's great.

898. It's hard to pick answers that pertain to every time I smoke, some days are different then others. I feel like a lot of people can be, and are responsible with their cannabis use, and then of course there are people that aren't and they are lazy and unmotivated and give the responsible smokers out there a bad name.

899. It's helped my headaches more than anything else. I've tried everything from going to a neurologist to acupuncture, massage, diet..,

900. It's helping me a lot and I am one of those conservative types that in the past would have never considered it, but glad I took the time to research my decision and give it a try.

901. It's important to distinguish between Regs and Krips because an 3.5 of regs is less than a gram of Krips and 1hit from Krips is equal to 4 or 5 hits from regs.

902. It's miraculous and beautiful. I support legalization and

personal freedom. I also support the full legalization of Kratom which is more medically useful for the treatment of abdominal / digestive tract pain in my experience than any other natural remedy or even changes in diet.

903. It's no better or worse than any other drug out there. But it is a gentle drug.

904. It's not addictive but some people might say it is but I have quit plenty of times for a month was the longest but I could go longer but I choose not to because I'm a happier person when I use it not just when I'm 'baked' but even when I haven't yet for the day. It's always nice to have something to look forward to after a long day of work.

905. It's not addictive.... It helps me be able to take my MS drugs. Helps me sleep. I was talking with my cos about her brother smoking and she said his babies, babies would have a birth defect... Lol.... Her mom smoked with her n her babies r fine... I just wanted to laugh.

906. It's peaceful, delightful and an alternative to so many proscription drugs. Legalize. peace.

907. It's really hard to say what the specific effects of cannabis is because of how sativa and indica both affect people in different ways. Sometimes when i smoke I want to draw and write and be creative and active and then at other times I just want to sit and watch tv and maybe talk.

908. It's ridiculous people can't smoke a joint but can go out and drink enough alcohol to not even be able to walk. Take it easy

909. Its about as awesome as Garlic

910. Its all on the strain and the different canainoids, Just because something has a high THC rating does't mean that it will effect you as well or as hard as something with a good blend of cannaoids. Different types and strains will effect people differently. One may put them to sleep while another my motivate them and engergize them. Just awesome.

911. its has really helped me thought some rough times and probably wouldn't be here if it wasn't for this miracle plant!

912. Its non addictive. It can be abused. But also does many people good. My use is rare due to the laws and current legal trouble due to Cannabis.

913. Its past time to make it legal for all over21. Medicaly for all ages, I personally wish there was more research done and less lies spread by are govt. What are we really missing from said drug

914. Its really hard to stop using it without becoming a bastard all of the time. my outlook on life is extremely poor in that im an absurdist, in the classical sense in which i view that lifes has no mening and we still search for one but that search is pointless yet we continue to look for an answer knowing that search is pointless. But ive had insomnia since i was 5 years old, i just can t sleep and i havent told doctors because i dont want ty damage my liver with pills and if i have them, i'll likely take them...mj has help me since freshman year in college fall asleep and rid crushing panic attacks induced by a micromanaging father who would disapprove 100 percent and the general

pressures of school. now im employed full time immediately out of college ilving alone leading a fully functional lifestyle. i smoke when i get home from work to fall asleep because it slows my busy brain.

915. its the healing of the nation, i plant out door thats the best not under artificial lights, if i would have more at my avail i would smoke more and make more products out of it like the oil, i also use seeds and leaves and roots

916. its the oldest medicine known to man other than ginger. its natural. I used to smoke it with tobacco mixed in with my joints for a smoother burn but i ended just getting addicted to the nicotine. If everyone had 10 minutes to themselves daily to smoke a joint - that small window for reflection (a mild meditation) would do the world some good. No deaths. side affects from weed i think come from those who have genial defects from alcohol abuse or certain illnesses. Im very lucky, no loss of motivation, since starting smoking my life has dramatically improved, I have had better jobs, better experiences, im surrounded my good people and friends. Weed smokers share haha unlike harder drug users who get possessive over their drugs. The amount of toxins are minimal of that compared to alcohol - I wonder why thats even still legal. I love you weed. X

917. Its the only thing that's helps the pain, sleep anxiety, life. Ive tried every medication under the sun. I used to believe its just people that wanted to get high, hell, i was getting high. but then i had the accident and everything changed.

918. ive had depression and severe anxiety since puberty; cannabis

use has since given me quality of life. i feel that it holds me back in life; not because of its effects, but due to its legal status(black market prices, no choice in strain and drastic variations in quality).

919. JUST FILED FOR MY CARD IN xx. I LISTENED TO THE xx AND AVOIDED CANNABIS IN ORDER TO GET THE PAIN MEDS I NEEDED. L5S1FUSED/ SIATICA/ T2HERNIATION/ MIGRANES/ MUSCLE SPASMS/ SHORTENED ULNA WITH 5IN PLATE AND 7 SCREWS/ 4 PINS FUSING WRIST/ HIGH BLOOD PSI/ LIVER ISSUES FROM OAPIATES/ MEMORY ISSUES FROM OAPIATES/ I just started cannabis seriously this summer (2014) first started about a year ago with GREAT HELP to almost all my issues. I finally had enough and tried it against the xx's policy. life was so bad i just had to try it and see if it even helped a little bit. IT HELPED LOTS! now after i told doc i did this she says xx will not stop my other meds due to cannabis use if im legal with a card. havent seen this happen yet, but dont trust them as far as i can throw them! I DONT CARE IT HELPS SO MUCH I HAVE TO!!!! and not even a high dose. i dont even get cotton mouth and red eyes. Using only at night for 2 weeks gave me results all day. made life better. GOAL: is to reduce oapiates and any other meds i can. i HATE the THC head high but ive gotten past it. I avoided my oxycodone cuz it tweaked my head. But this i control better. slowly titrating levels up comfortable. vaporizer helps do that well. EX: bag from vape with pinch of cannabis (barely any vapor) and wait 10 min. again if needed. I just found an indica for night sleep and pain. I got 2.5hours of straight sleep. no flopin, no urge to piss, and my day was SO much better the next day with just more sleep. I didnt feel drugged like the sleeping pills and no FOG the next day like the pills do! My name is xxx, you can send me questionares or questions to xxxxxxxxxxxxxxxxxx

920. just one thing to add, sometimes when i'm high, i'm able to really focus and immerse myself in doing something. That could be sports, art, whatever. I just tend to completely focus on that one thing, and with everything, including sports, I've seen no negative impacts on my performance

921. Just that it should be totally legal, it harms no one if used responsibly.

922. Keep medical marijuana program separate from recreational so I can continue to be able to grow my own thus being able to afford the medication that helps me survive the pain I endure

923. Keep on keepin' on.

924. Keep up the good work!

925. Keep up the good work.

926. Kill the republicans

927. know that on the drinking question, i binge drink on friday and saturday nights, and then don't drink at all during the week

928. Knowing the exact THC level is a big help because dosing is predictable and repeatable. That has been a big step forward. We need a lot more research into Cannabis chemistry and pharmacology. It would be nice to have some means of getting a dose rapidly without smoking or vaping. Sublingual absorption of tincture does not seem to work. I haven't tried rectal administration. ;)

929. l have smoked off & on & grown my own ~ only in the last couple of years did I start again after my mother died on our front lawn we started smoking ~ ionly in the last 6 months did I find out just how amzing this plant is ~ I would really love to juice it ~ but you need so many plants ~ god bless

930. Legal acrossed the US

931. LEGALISE CANNABIS! Regulate like alcohol

932. Legalise it

933. Legalise it soon as, more medical investigation into its benifits.

934. Legalization needs to happen

935. Legalize

936. Legalize it!

937. legalize it!

938. Legalize it! Daily user and my only stress in life is that my pot is illegal!

939. legalize it!!!!!!!

940. Legalize it.

941. Legalize it.

942. Legalize it. I shouldnt have to fear going to jail because I choose

to medicate my self. I was on prescriptions that were addictive and had to go through withdrawals to get off of. That is crazy. I will never allow a doctor to prescribe me medication again.

943. Legalize it. It's time.

944. Legalize the weed let people grow there own without fear of going to prison.

945. Legalize this shit!!!

946. Legalize world wide as the war on drugs will never be won and also incarcerates too many innocent recreational users.

947. Legalized, lightly taxed. Anti-cancer properties need to be scientifically tested and explored incredibly thoroughly. No permits should be required to grow your own plants. Homegrown should have no government interference, or distribution of homegrown. Penalties only when distributing to those underage.

948. Let people smoke it and tax it then everyone will win. Cannabis is only bad if you abuse it, just like drinking.....

949. Let's regulate a natural plant that has caused no deaths in its record of existence. It may be a factor in the onset of psychosis but only to those who have a prior disposition to the illness.

950. Like everything else, it is not for everyone and affects every person differently.

951. Living in WA state as a medicinal patient it is very concerning that they are now trying to eliminate medicinal cannabis entirely,

simply over the fact the state makes at a minimum double with the recreational stores over the medical dispensaries. There are many patients simply too sick to go deal with the hassles of a recreational pot store - between the long lines & they sell out frequently how is THAT helpful? as more specialized cannabis products are developed I am finding I am smoking flower less and less. Why can't recreational sales be restricted to FLOWER ONLY? Leave the mmj dispensaries alone - I know before I had my mmj authorization and was using cannabis occasionally simply for the 'high' I smoked flower - recreational users don't need RSO oil - high CBD vape cartridges or transdermal patches - that is just ONE idea, I imagine there are thousands of other ideas out there that may be a better solution

952. luck good.

953. Majority of those that I know who use it recreational are actually using it for medical related reasons. Not all conditions are covered by medical marijuana states, such as Washington does not cover Crohn's Disease as a condition considered for MMJ.

954. Make it legal and save lives:-):-):-)

955. many of the answers to your questions would vary depending upon the dosage, or quantity/potency of the cannabis consumed.

956. Many of the most intelligent, most athletic, most productive people I know are regular cannabis users. There's nothing I can tell you haven't already heard. Thank you for doing this research.

957. Many of the myths surrounding Cannabis use are unfounded and false. For example, that Cannabis immediately urges one to eat junk food snacks... That Cannabis makes one stupid and confused... That using it makes one lazy and lethargic. For me, using Cannabis raises my level of the perception of beauty and harmony. It increases my awareness of the spiritual side of life, gets me in tune with my body, eases tension and allows me to step back from the frantic pace of modern life.

958. Many of the short-term effects differ on a session by session basis or by method/

959. Many users of cannabis, myself including, read and do our best to understand the interaction of cannabinoids and the endocannabinoid system. I have spent a lot of time growing to find a sativa leaning pheno with high CBD. It's lucid, mildly euphoric with high pain relief. I have other plant's for specific pain, specific effects. High amounts of euclyptol, a terpene, helps greatly with my asthma. THCV when in combination with CBG dilates my vein, lowering my blood pressure, and allowing better oxygen saturation (I have Mediterranean anemia as well). I hope that well informed patients such as myself will continue to be able to explore which strains were best myself, and that control doesn't move into the hands of a few company, which I fear, would lead to very few conditions truly being well met.

960. Many years years ago, I was a heavy alcohol binge drinker, a meth addict, and smoked 2 packs of cigarettes/ day. During that time, I did not use Cannabis regularly. When I first stopped using the other substances, I did use Cannabis more frequently. However, it never controlled my life, nor has it

ever been the focus of my choices the way that the addictive substances were. Now I use it more for a specific purpose such as insomnia or headaches, and less for recreation. This has been a natural evolution rather than a conscious decision. I have also found that the same dose works just as effectively regardless of how often I use or don't use. This is the opposite of addictive substances.

961. Marijauna is a miracle drug, it can cure many ailments including cancer ...the fda should pull there heads out of their asses and start curing cancer rather than treating it with experimental drugs that are ruining peoples bodys and lives and costing billions of dollars in the process

962. Marijuana changed my life for the better. I can't even describe how much happier, calmer, more empathetic, patient, and overall much nicer than I was before I started. I love it.

963. marijuana free my mind

964. Marijuana has changed my life and I am so grateful to that little plant! I feel safe in a state that allows me to use Cannabis to treat myself. I do not drive under the influence as a rule.

965. Marijuana has helped relieve my generalized anxiety helping tremendously with the stomach problems that crippled my high school years. I attend a great college where many people smoke and yet my stats is without medical or decrim. I love the plant and it's helped me a lot.

966. Marijuana has opened my mind and allowed me to spend time within myself for deep contemplative soul work. It increases my

awareness of my surroundings. Colors are more vivid. Being in nature makes you feel even more at peace. I experience profound revelations about my personal relationships and goals in life, which stick with me beyond the high. I feel more spiritual and more self aware and am very lucky to have experienced this herb at the age I have. Too much of anything is bad, but small doses of marijuana occasionally can have amazing eye opening experiences that can alter your perception of daily life.

967. Marijuana has transformed my life. Coupled with several other drastic life chsnges, my quality of life has improved exponentially. I am more motivated, more fit and I have marijuana to thank for having fscilitated such change.

968. Marijuana helps me connect with nature. It gives me a brand new perspective and respect for everything. It also makes everything look a little more beautiful. It's like putting goggles that filter all the bad out of the world.

969. marijuana if used chronically (1-6days a week) has had a negative impact on my life. Marijuana is great when your tolerance is low and you can smoke as much as you drink. Certainly smoking chronically is nowhere near as bad as drinking chronically in my experience, but there is a detrimental effect....tiredness when sober, loss of motivation, problems receiving dopamine for positive actions. It's safer than alcohol but should not be seen as an ideal way to get through life.

970. Marijuana is a good healing medication for anyone with chronic pain.

971. Marijuana is a good way to calm down and relieve stress.

972. Marijuana is a verry critica component of my spiritual life. I believe people should be more aware of the positive mental and spiritual effects of marijuana.

973. Marijuana is an amazing effective drug but the same with everything moderation is key

974. Marijuana is definitely not physically additive but it can become a bad habit especially when I use it as an escape route to calm down. Weed neither improves or decreases my motivation. I will have the same motivational issues with or without smoking. and I don't drive.

975. Marijuana is not an addictive thing. It's associated with bad drugs because it's illegal. It has helped me be able to eat and not hurt after eating. Also your questions were really contradicting. When I do not smoke I feel anxiety but it's not due to not smoking or withdrawals. I felt the anxiety before. Marijuana helps me calm it down.

976. Marijuana is safer than any antidepressant I have been prescribed. It has fewer to no side affects unlike man made pills. The reasons for prohibition of marijuana in the USA have nothing to do with the safety of consuming the plant, but are based primarily on money. It should definitely not be a schedule one drug since the US federal government supplies marijuana to four citizens for medicinal reasons.

977. Marijuana is the only reason i was able to control and then quit a heroin addiction. I did it without going into any kind of rehab. Just weed and talking to a psychologist. I smoked copious amounts all day long and it was able to sooth out most of the

withdrawal symptoms and then cravings I would get. Because of all of this, though (I believe), when I don't smoke for more than 1 day the withdrawals I get feel far worse than anyone else I've ever talked to about weed withdrawals. When I was in high school, and before I had ever done any hard drugs, I could smoke 30 days straight and then stop for a week and not feel any withdrawals at all.

978. Marijuana makes me quite itchy one hour after smoking, particularly with indica dominant strains.

979. Marijuana saved my life. I was on 16 different drugs and day from my Dr's and those drugs were killing me. I was 130 pounds overweight and could barely get out of bed. Now I have lost weight and feel like a human being again. The only medicine I take is synthroid and marijuana.

980. Marijuana seems to magnify/accent the state you are in already... If you are already anxious/ nervous, it can accent that. You can use it to clean your house (motivate), or you can use it to relax.

981. Marijuana should be legalized so there can be different/safer ways to consume the medicine part of it.

982. Measure cannabis usage and ability to function at work.

983. Medical cannabis allows me to function when my stomach issues are otherwise debilitating. I take a low enough dose for symptom treatment that I feel no psychoactive, but significant physical, effects.

984. Medical Cannabis has been life changing with chronic pain! CBD was an amazing discovery!

985. Medical cannabis has changed my life by making my chronic pain from previous soft tissue injuries, fibromyalgia, arthritis, menstrual cramps, and even typical occasional pain (e.g. dental issues, sprains) far more tolerable. Higher CBD strains have a positive effect on my pain and inflammation, even the following day or two. It's had a positive effect on my moods, behaviors, and even lingering PTSD issues. I've lost 60+ pounds over the past year because cannabis has made it tolerable to move and exercise more and eat healthy foods more frequently, which has a positive effect on my blood sugar (I also have hypothyroidism and PCOS). I'm a stay-at-home-mom for a 4-xxxxxxxxx with High Functioning Autism, so not really unemployed, more like employed 24/7. A month ago, I was forced to STOP cannabis when xxxxxxxxxxxxxxxxx xxxxxxxxxxxx took over the pain clinic I was receiving excellent care from xxxxxx's policy is to not prescribe opioids for patients using cannabis. Sadly, I need both medications right now to function, but I hope to continue to reduce the oxycodone and only use cannabis at some point. I'm only at 50% function of where I was a month or two ago, when I could medicate with cannabis as needed. Anyway, I hope this study helps change the minds and policies of many doctors, particularly those who deal with chronic pain. I've found that even general practitioners who fully believe in the healing properties of cannabis are often handcuffed by the anti-cannabis policies of their practices and/or fears of DEA retribution. Thanks for studying this important topic!

986. Medical Cannabis use has been life changing for me. I was in a car accident in 2011 and was resigned to taking opiates for the rest of my life, to cover up the pain. This became a problem because your body gets used to opiates. So, in my case, in two and a half years, I went from Tylenol 3 to Morphine. On top of

this, I was having to take several other medications, to attempt to deal with the side effects of the opiates. This cocktail left me unable to care for myself, in even some of the most basic ways. Cannabis was a Godsend. I had never smoked pot, but it really felt like my last hope for medication that wasn't going to destroy my body. It's lived up to my expectations and then some. I was able to get off the opiates, over two years ago, and I've never looked back. Not only was I able to stop taking opiates, but also all the other horrible medications that I had to take because of them too. The 'Western Medication' messed up my digestion worse than I could have imagined. I've spent the past two years working on healing it and I have Cannabis to thank for beginning that journey. In addition to my body operating much better on Cannabis vs. opiates, my brain does too. When I was taking opiates, I had no hope of ever going back to work, even to something simple and part time. Now, as I continue to slowly improve, the world is starting to feel like my oyster. I hope that one day I can use my experience as a patient with chronic pain to help others. I know this study is just about usage, but I also want to make the statement that I think it's poor legislation to combine medical dispensaries and recreational stores. From my perspective, the medical patient and the recreational client are looking to make very different purchases. My understanding is that the sole purpose of smoking recreationally is to get high. As a medical patient, that is not my sole purpose and what each patient is looking for varies based on their condition. They look for different application/usage/ingestion methods, strains, and various ratios of THC and CBD. My fear is that combining it all into one industry will kill the variety that the medical dispensaries once possessed, making them a far less valuable resource.

987. Medical cannibus products are able to effectively treat a wide range ofconditions that most recreational form marijuana would be to dumbed down to even touch... research Simpson oil and how it affected we stopping cancer in its tracks... these are one of the many necessary medicines that would become illegal under the new 502 initiative!! pretty much anything that could effectively treat any kind of actual medical condition would not be sold or available under a recreational tyranee!! patients in my state were told that I 502 would not affect medical marijuana or its laws.. now that the Liquor Control Board has control of it as a citizen's initiative they are trying to remove all patients rights that we have had for 15 years in Washington! they want to make a mockery of marijuana.. Force medical patients into a 502 market completely eliminating self propagation of all forms! this is a travesty!! they want to amend the laws in RCW 6951 a the tie them to the new 502 laws that way when the time comes they can sink them both with the same torpedo.... probably sell low quality factory produced sativa that makes people drool on themselves... that way they can point fingers laugh and say ' just look what marijuana does to the people!'

988. Medical marijuana should be kept as a separate entity from recreational use. Please do what you can to keep this medicine for those of us that need it and have the option to grow a few plants for our own use.

989. medical marijuana should be made legal in all states for those with legitimate medical issues. It greatly helps to control my pain and suffering. Much better than prescription drugs.

990. Medical needs differ from the desires of recreational users. Medical users need consistent quality of the strains that work for

them. They often need need larger amounts and take cannabis in multiple forms I used edibles, capsules and vaporization. Each form has advantages for the medical user.

991. Medical professional. Regulation needed. Many people use for medical reasons , safety and respect should be used and considerd

992. Medically: Cannabis has helped me relieve pain (while remaining functional), reduce anxiety (without addiction issues like Xanax/Ativan), alleviate my depression (without side effects of weight gain, loss of sex drive, paradoxical suicidal ideation, or the 'foggy-head' feeling), and help counter-act the side effects associated with my Lithium. Recreational: I feel that a lot of the recreational value of marijuana probably helps me out medically. Getting high as fuck, stoned off my ass blazed keeps me level-headed, helps me sleep, helps me write, helps me get over my depression which helps me become more attentive to my significant other. Now, just smoking a little bit can do wonders for me as well. Big project I need to get done? 1-2 quick hits off a bowl and I'm good to go. It can also help you unwind after an especially irritating day, but without all of the dangers that come with other potential drugs.

993. Might be interesting to ask questions around common activities people engage in while using it.

994. Missing in how you select your cannabis is how I select mine - try it - didn't work, move on to the next one until I find those that work. Under driving, you didn't allow for those of us who don't drive - I don't. Family income doesn't make good sense without knowing how many in the family and many won't

answer that one, anyway. Finally, if you're going to ask about substance abuse history, you need to ask how long ago - I've been clean for 40 years!

995. Mmj is the best med known to man. Contact me if you want my full story from age of7months

996. More effective and less down side than ANY anti depressant or pain killer. Best MEDICINE for a variety of symptoms I have ever used.

997. More research need to be done on the many benefits of cannabis.

998. More research needs to be done to show the medical benefits of cannabis.

999. Most of my friends and work colleagues all smoke weed. Some are college educated, some blue collar workers. The one thing I can say about weed smokers is that they get up and go to work everyday. They take care of their responsibilities first and smoking is just a way to relax or a hobby. I know plenty of regular smokers who have to pass a drug test for work, or a new job and just quit smoking the month before with no problem. Then they either stay smoke free, or go back until they have to pass another test. Most of the young professionals I know who smoke have never done any other drugs or used tobacco regularly. I think the persecution of cannabis users is absurd. Right now NH is trying to pass a legalization law for recreational use. I doubt it will pass this year, but I hope it does and I honestly think that within 10 years weed will be legal all over the US because when you really look around, there are tons of closet smokers, or people who would smoke if it was legal.

1000. Most of the reason that I use cannabis is recreational--it helps take the edge off of anxiety, especially when I'm experiencing trauma activation. That having been said, I have also worked with a lot of clients (as an herbalist, nutritionist) who used cannabis all day every day, and I believe it was deleterious to their wellbeing, just as drinking all day every day might be...

1001. Mostly helps me relax from a long day at work.

1002. Mostly use low THC dose pretzels to relax. They travel well. If I smoke it's maximum 1 or 2 puffs in a pipe as its so potent these days.

1003. Must educate. Everyone uses Cannabid for a readon. Important to knoe what that reason is. Thanks :)

1004. My answer to 'IN THE PAST 7 DAYS..... How often have you been bothered by emotional problems such as feeling anxious, depressed or irritable?' Is because of stress which has nothing to do with a consumption of cannabis.

1005. my answers as to how often I use cannabis is based soley on availability and cost. If I could legally use and afford cannabis for my pain management, insomnia, depression, (instead of pharmaceutical drugs), I would surely do so.

1006. My brother overused cannabis at, what i consider, a very young age, 14. I feel that using cannabis at this young can alter and affect your brain and should not be used. I started using cannabis at 18 and i feel that is the perfect age as you have more of an understanding and maturity and are able to think for yourself more. I feel that cannabis should legalised and controlled in the same way we use alcohol. We had a similar problem in the 1920's with alcohol bootlegging and we managed to solve that in that era. Now that we are in a much more technologically and socially advanced ciommunity, why are we struggling so much to eliminate the problems which illegalisation causes. The more things outlaws, the more outlaws run!

1007. My Cannabis use affects no one, it does not stop me from achieving anything, if it did I would stop taking it. Cannabis needs to be legal in the world now.

1008. My cannabis use has changed over time. While I used to use it more recreationally, I now use cannabis with intention; whether it be for creative inspiration, connection in nature, increased body awareness and healing, or meditation. This is common for many cannabis users I know who have a long history of use. The effects of cannabis on my body are wide-ranging, for example while sometimes it can increase my desire to eat, it also instills a profound consciousness of how I am feeling in my body, which often produces the opposite effect (I realize my body is in its digesting phase and has no need for food). I do believe the ritual/act of cannabis can be addictive, but the plant itself is not. Thank you!

1009. My cannabis use has seemed to be a roller coaster ride over the past three years. Going to college and leaving my home town, meeting new people, the challenges of being on my own were all hard things to do. Sometimes I think using cannabis helped those times, either alone or with friends and new people. I think in the long run, cannabis helped my social health, but my mental and body health may be implicated. I definitely experience long term memory loss, and sometimes I feel like

I am addicted to the drug. But I still feel that it helps me with my anxiety, and I don't think I will stop using it. I have learned to control my use of cannabis, and I feel like I could stop and be totally fine cutting cold turkey, which I have done several times in the past. I choose to recreationally use the drug the same way a family comes together over a meal, or the same way someone might watch TV or calm down in the nighttime on their own. I would say cannabis has improved my quality of life, but some of the physical health and cognitive defects may hurt me in the long run.

1010. My epilepsy medication makes me severely depressed. I also get high anxiety from it. Cannabis helps with all of my medication side effects. I have recently significantly decreases my epilepsy medication and am using a keto diet, naturopathic recommendations and medications as well as cannabis to control my seizures. I love cannabis but I dislike being stoned all day so I only start smoking mid afternoon on. My care provider grows me a high CBD strain and this is the most medicinal for my epilepsy. If I could find a CBD only strain I would smoke all day. However the TCH is what helps with my anxiety and my lack of appetite problems so I do have a high TCH strain to smoke right before dinner and right before bed. I hope this helps!

1011. my experiences vary - meaning that sometimes I smoke more or sometimes I smoke less. Money determines a lot of my use decisions. I use a lot topically and have found this really helps with pain and headaches. I'm going to try suppositories for my IBS now that I've heard they are available.

1012. My family only uses cannabis medicinally for asthma and pain related problems. We do not use it recreationally. Just to bathe or soak in cannabis or drink a teaspoon of a tonic made from soaking cannabis buds and leaves in rum.

1013. My general health and motivation scores are much lower than they would be as I was diagnosed with ulcerative colitis not too long ago. In have been exposed to cannabis my whole life and do not believe that, in moderation, it is at all harmful. I have not tried it as a treatment for my current condition. Although, I have been told it work great for crones.

1014. My girlfriend and I work freelance in several creative industries ranging from photography to video and animation as well as branding and web design. We work all day everyday and usually smoke towards the end of the day. I have a hard time 'turning my mind off' and often have several tedious tasks to take care of regularly. I also have insomnia and depression. Smoking makes all those things a little more tolerable and is something I enjoy. My girlfriend has bad social anxiety and it helps her in large groups and when she gets overwhelmed with work it helps her focus on what she needs to get done. I know it's not great for my lungs and we try to vape as much as possible but it does effect you differently.

1015. My husband and I are both regular, daily users in a state where medicinal use is illegal. We excel in corporate, stressful jobs, own our home and maintain great relationships with friends and family. We do have problems cutting down and use it to unwind in the evenings, like having a glass of wine.

1016. My interest in mmj is for my young daughter who has severe epilepsy. I have only used cannabis myself to see how her mess could potentially affect her.

1017. My life turned around once I started using cannabis. Before I had anger issues, PTSD due to be raped at age 6, and suffered from major depression. I was never hungry and didn't not like what I saw when I looked in the mirror. Cannabis changed my life around. I eat a healthy diet with no depression or Ptsd problems. I have more energy to do what needs done and I make friends alot more easy. I have never had any problems with cannabis and would be far off worse if I hadn't tried it. The medicine I was being prescribed only made my symptoms worse which is when I found out cannabis made things better. LEGALIZE IN ALL 50 STATES!!!!

1018. My lung collapsed last year (spontaneous neuxmothorax). I had been smoking quite heavily up till then. Used a vapourizer for up to year after but have returned to joints now, although not as much as before. I also have coeliac disease and oral allergy syndrome.

1019. My major complaint is ongoing arthritic and fibromyalgia pain. Using cannabis, via vaporization, removes the pain quickly and gives me approx 2 hours of relief. Prior to using cannabis, I was 'huffing and puffing in pain' around mid-afternoon every day. My pain level / inflammation is much reduced, with arthritic pain peaking in the late afternoon/ evening. I now vaporize in the evenings. I found that my ADD (inattenitive type) is reduced in impact when I use specific Sativa and sativa-dominant hybrid strains. I also found that some strains are excellent for sleep, others for creativity. Now with the Washington state dispensary laws changed, I find that I am needing a whole new system for getting Rx for cannabis use. This is a frustrating and irritating thing for me. My MD is supportive, but the healthcare cooperative does not authorize such prescriptions. Therefore my health insurance does not cover the medical reference, so I have to establish new patient relationship with another provider. This is a financial burden for me.

1020. My mental health has been generally poor in the past, including multiple years of taking antidepressants, moderate to heavy alcohol intake as well as having to take benzodiazapines for anxiety. Since I have moved to Washington, where cannabis is legal I have been off of all prescription drugs and drink about 1/5 less than I did before having access to medical cannabis. I strongly prefer high CBD or equal ratio THC/CBD. I have noticed less impariment while smoking this kind versus smoking high THC variety. I have also noticed the short term memory loss is completely gone when smoking an equal ratio variety. High THC variety is a bit too intense and anxiety producing whereas the equal ratio kind is very anxiolytic, calming and also basically eliminates any depression which I previously experienced. High THC variety increased libido pretty strongly and also sensations, whereas the equal mix appears to be neutral. Another main reason I use cannabis is because of a sleep disorder that I have. I don't know if it is a real 'disorder', but I sleep very shallow and have continuous vivid dreams that seem real. They are not nightmares but boring and mundane activities that occur in them. I wake up feeling like I never went to sleep and exhausted. When I smoke a few hits of cannabis before bed it completely eliminates this excessive dreaming and I get sounder sleep and thus have improved energy during the day. This plant has changed my life or may even go so far as to say that it has saved my life.

1021. My pain & sleep are not regular & relieved with inhalation.

ADHD & appetite suppression are more chronic so I use edibles & tinctures.

1022. My pain was unbearable and the opiates are addictive. NSAIDs only tear up my stomach. My anxiety with people or in groups is highly diminished.

1023. My parents started me at age two. I have showed a loss in motivation on doing basic things. My memory seems to be fine, I surprise people on the crap I remember. I use it now mostly out of habit, but it does help with stress and anxiety. But I figure if alcohol and tobacco are legal, a substance that can cure cancers should be.

1024. My primary use of cannabis is for better sleep. I do not use it during my work day, and sometimes recreationally on weekends if I have no responsibilities to be carried out.

1025. My PTSD symptoms have improved dramatically in the past 6 months, since using a cbd heavy strain. I feel healthier, less anxious and more productive with the dosage I currently take.

1026. My quality of life has improved drastically I was very depressed had no motivation was a hikimori. Now I can just be y'know.

1027. My recreational use is often in response to minor pains and health issues, as well as anxiety and stress. I take no other medication for these issues. I however use about 2 times a day, regardless of medical needs because it is also recreational as well as addictive.

1028. My use is limited to the time after work and prior to going to sleep. I do not smoke when working, and that's where I tend toward irritability. I do not smoke to get stoned, in fact, I don't like being stoned. Treatment for substance abuse was specific to alcohol and cocaine, and I have been free of those substances for 28 years.

1029. My use of cannabis started out with medical purposes. Since I do not drink, I started looking at cannabis to see if it would be a viable recreational thing. I totally enjoy it in that capacity. Something else is I have quit smoking cigarettes for six months now. I seemed to have also found more pleasure in smoking cannabis rolled into joints. Just like a cigarette. Now when I consider the thought or attempt to quit smoking cannabis, my mind starts acting like it did when I started to quit cigarettes. Food for thought. Thank you

1030. Natural Organic Plants should not be illegal in a free society!

1031. Needs to be prove safe and effective

1032. Never asked for substance treatment. Was hospitalized and recommended so tried but had already quit at that point. Resumed use again after long time without due to stress and desire to relax.

1033. never used drugs in my life, this topical salv works where others didn't to relieve - hives, & excessively dry skin patch, allowing my hair to grow back

1034. Nice survey. I would reconsider how you word the question about 'how do you feel when your stoned' i took it as stoned from smoking indica. Stoned doest always describe every high. But thats a tricky situation. Glad i could participate.

1035. No one should have to suffer needlessly. If cannabis helps then so be it. Money should never stand in the way of easing the suffering of others.

1036. Nobody talks about using marijuana to treat bipolar disorder. To me it smooths out my highs and lows even when smoking only once or twice a week. I also believe it is addictive, but in the same way video games, sex, or gambling can be addictive, not like opiates or cocaine.

1037. not at all harmful , far better than prescription drugs

1038. Not half as bad as alcohol! Might be psychologically addictive for some people.

1039. Not much to say other than that it seems obvious that Cannabis has a lot to offer by way of medical usage and recreational and the industrial uses really need to be embraced as well. The industrial uses which allow for sustainable and renewable cultivation could really help reduce our reckless use of fossil fuels.

1040. Not only would cannabis legalization help with thousands of people 'breaking the law' every day but cannabis comes with hemp and hemp can be used for anything: plastic, clothes, paper, oil, etc. Cannabis is a billion dollar industry. We need to get on it!

1041. Note- for the 'how do you select your marijuana' question, there should be an 'I don't' option. That is, those of us not living in legal states take whatever's avalable. My dealer has one strain of weed, called 'weed'.

1042. Nothing wrong with sparking up a bowl after a long day. I feel that cannabis is a pair of glasses I can put on that lets me see the world clearly.

1043. Occasional User, receive from individuals who have medical marijuana cards.

1044. On the short term questionnaire, I had to answer both ways on some since different buds can have different effects.

1045. Once I realized that all of the prescriptions that was on had a side effect of death, and especially at the doses I was taking due to tolerance and metabolic issues, there was no other choice for me. And since switching to a natural medicine, my joints feel better than they have in years. I think the pharma was causing a portion of the pain, or the cannabis is just that good, either way, I can't go back!

1046. Once you have started increasing usage/dosage per week, it's hard to stop, and I can personally attest to that. That's where my view of it as 'addictive' comes from.

1047. One medical use not listed is for coughs. When I have the cold/flu and get a dry, unproductive cough, running a bag-style vaporizer through a water pipe is really useful in loosening up my cough and making other acute symptoms less painful.

1048. Only creating criminals out of innocent people since 1937! Pharmaceuticals is a 400 billion dollar per year industry, yet what happens here in America every 19 minutes? Google it! It is also known for as a cure for many many many different things. Just think that it could do to the economy? Saving millions upon millions per day/week/moth/year and state incarcerating pedifiles with victims than one who is the victim to a plant. Provided by from who ever it is up above.... I am a convicted felon from Cannabis! I refused 3yrs on papers and served 6 months in prison! And got smoked out while in prison and once I got picked up at the front gate the day of my release! Only thing dangerous about it, is getting caught!

1049. Only effective drug from sever anxiety with related depression, as well as severe IBS. I have seen doctors but the process of getting a medical marijuana card is too much trouble under the Harper government for it to be worth all the time and money. Just a big scam. Honestly, I have reduced all drug use from ibuprofen to prescriptions once I started self-medicating with cannabis.

1050. Opiates stole my early twenties. Cannabis gave me back my late twenties. I also do not believe I would have ever conceived my daughter if not for my constant consumption - I had pre-cancerous cysts covering my ovaries and was told from age 14 that I was most likely barren due to it. At age 29, after absolutely no life changes except the exclusion of opiates and inclusion of cannabis, I conceived my daughter. I was later told that there were no abnormalities whatsoever in my ovaries. The doctors seemed hesitant to attribute it to cannabis therapy, but I am absolutely certain that without it, I would have never had what I wanted (and now treasure) most in the world.

1051. Our endocannabinoid system is crucial to our health and cannibis is wonderful at stimulating this system I have seen so many 'miracles' from cannabis, and it needs to be harnessed.

1052. Out off all the drugs I have taken and there has been alot cannabis is the safest and the lest drug I have had problems with the only 2 things I can personally say is how addited I am to every day use and the money I am spending on my use a week ex: over Â£200. Cannabis should be made legal for medical and recreation world wide. People wake up a relise that what you think you know about cannabis is most probably wrong

1053. Over the years, I've learned that smaller doses of cannabis provide more favorable states of being, ie. feel like stretching/ exercising, creative and alternative perspectives on things, less paranoia/anxiety, general feeling of well-being.

1054. Patients must be allowed to continue growing their own medicine. Patients have been growing their own medicine for over 15yrs & without the right to grow their own medicine many patients would not be able to afford the medicine they need to keep them alive. I'm sorry if our (patients) being sick isn't convenient for those trying to start a recreational marijuana market but our need is one of necessity, not recreational use. Medical & recreational must remain separate programs, which is what the people of Washington State voted for when we approved RCW 69.51 et al. Patients were lied to by the authors & supporters of I-502 when they claimed that the passing of I-502 would not affect or interfere with medical marijuana, now they want to throw patients under the bus, end the medical marijuana programs, eliminate patients right to grow their own medicine & set highly restrictive quantity limits. When prepapring Concentrates like Cannabis Oil, it takes far more than the three ounce quantity limit proposed by the Washington State Liquor Control Board hearing last night, 11/13/2013. There are so many more problems with the planned implementation of I-502, more than I could hope to fit in this space, one of the biggest concerns is the allegations that many people have been allowed to buy the recreational marijuana business licenses that aren't supposed to be available until AFTER I-502 is implemented, for a $20,000 cash payment! The Washington State Patrol has been made aware of these allegations & has been asked to investigate, as far as I know, no investigation has been iniated as of my composing this message. I believe the Attorney General's Office has also been asked to investigate these allegations, along with allegations of corruption by Washington's Governor. Thank you for taking the time to circulate this survey, medical marijuana is medicine & many patient's lives depend on their being able to have safe access to it.

1055. Patients must be allowed to grow their own in their garden and not go to jail in Canada.

1056. people around hge world is abused by police for using cannabis...they dont care..they just use as a weapon against u..usa is responsable of the war against cannabis..so..time to say sorry to the world..legalize it..its just a plant..better 1 milion st...oners then a single bad corrupted police guy...

1057. People should know the pros AND the cons of medical marijuana. Most users are blind to the cons. Most non-users are blind to the pros. Not a great learning system thus the overreactions to a relatively benign drug and under-reactions to whatever harms it does pose.

1058. People smoke weed in other states too....

1059. People who use cannabis, often do so because they don't believe there is any real danger to do so responsibly.

1060. Perhaps have a section asking people to identify problems they are aware of to do with cannabis consumption, ie smoke inhalation, getting mentally addicted (not physically) etc.

1061. Please, make sure, they legalise it, thank you for doing good work :)

1062. Politicians and Corporations are lying to the American public and/or they are ignorant about how beneficial marijuana is and its effects on a person's spiritual, physical and mental states. It is sad that with all the new and past studies on marijuana, that our federal and (most) our state governments are either ignorant or worst yet, financially motivated to not legalize marijuana like they have alcohol. As a result, I don't trust these 'leaders.' Why can my government say that something that God created is illegal? God made every seed bearing plant for our good...and what God creates (unlike a lot of humans...in my opinion) is good!

1063. post a link to this survey on www.reddit.com/r/trees

1064. Pot can be a very positive force in someone's life or it have a negative impact. It is up to each user to control their consumption. If I smoke too often, I will experience depression for about a week when I stop.

1065. Pot is far less harmful in every way than alcohol and thus should be fully legal throughout the world. A beautiful lifestyle can be created with a few hits a day. Allows you to 'not sweat the small stuff' as much! Also, as a Type A personality, it mitigates my over- controlling and bossy behavior, so I use it as a mood stabilizer, and a 'witness' to my unwanted antisocial tendencies.

1066. Pot is not the boogie man it's been portrayed as. Most people would not have a problem consuming it.

1067. Pot should be cheaper for students

1068. Prefer the term social to recreational. For me cannabis use seems to have helped me stay healthy, no prescription drugs, no cancer, no heart issues. Not saying there is a connection but those are the facts.

1069. Pretty my pot habit saved my life. I was really ridiculously high strung before, and pot helped put my world into perspective and helped me prioritize my activities

1070. Proper dosage and Quality Control (in the cannabis production Industry) is extremely important to me as a cannabis enjoyer.

1071. Pushing the state to legalize cannabis will prove to be a big mistake in my opinion. Over-regulation and excessive taxation will occur, making it harder for peaceful stoners, and sick/ suffering cannabis patients alike to obtain quality medicine at a reasonable cost. The state liquor board is an overbearing extortionist agency that charges a %72.4 tax *in addition to* 20.47 cents/liter on liquor. Liquor is a luxury item. The tax is quite high, but it's not going to hurt anyone that can't afford it. Cannabis is a powerful medicine that can heal disease and mitigate suffering in the seriously ill, and the cannabis community at large has foolishly begged to have the state to tax and control it. I can only pray that the state will not impose the heavy taxes that it has with alcohol.

1072. Quality of the product along with chemical constituents are huge players in the flower world for me. If too many chemicals (prefer organic) are used during the grow of cannabis, my conditions worsen.

1073. Questions could yield much more useful data with helpful collaboration between Bastyr research staff, and cannabis industry veterans. Questions like how much does one consume, is impossible to answer if individuals are exclusively oil users. Questions about RSO would yield startling differences across age groups. In general, there are dozens of tweaks, or additional questions that would allow for your research staff to get a more complete picture of how cannabis, in all it's forms, can interact with individuals on average. Good luck!

1074. Raw cannabis juice is very underestimated use of cannabis. Why don't doctors get a better understanding on what they are recommending? People that work at medical cannabis sites should have better training. A Bastyr approved Cannabis class for all doctors giving recommendations and staff of Medical approved facilities.

1075. Really helps a lot of people, myself included. Truly an effective medicine.

1076. Recently eating a sm amount of cannabus made me feel extremly anxious and a fast heart beat (last time i checked it at rest was 110 bpm) this lasts 2-4 hrs. I am now afraid to eat medicated edibles and will prob never try it again because i had such a bad experience. in the past it i never had a bad exp. Only in the past 4 months did it ever bother me (3x).

1077. Recreation use of cannabis is recommended. However, very frequent use will change life-style. Less, and less-serious, side-effects than alcohol by a huge margin. Far more socially-integrative than any other substance I know of - and I have tried many - both prescribed and illegal. Grass more conducive to pleasurable effects than solids.

1078. Recreational and medical marijuana are two different subjects and should be treated as such. The two areas should never overlap, patients should be allowed their privacy by allowing them access to dispensaries while recreational users should get their cannabis from retail stores only. Regulation for both fields should not be bundled together whatsoever.

1079. recreational cannabis has similar intoxication and physiological efects of coffee. it works as a neuro modulator

1080. Recreational cannabis use is not always linked with a desire to experience delirious and disconnecting effects.

1081. recreational use is often actual medicinal use, to relieve stress, expand thinking, obtain relief from societal dronishness, etc. Smoking anything is harmful because of heat applied directly to sensitive body tissues in mouth throat & lungs. Some vaporizers even produce 300 degree (Fahrenheit) smoke

1082. Recreationally I smoke maybe once every 2-3 months. I have 2 major back surgeries in less than a year and live in chronic, severe pain - nerve damage has left me unable to sit, stand, walk or even lie down comfortably for more than 20-30 minutes. I wake often at night from the pain. I have an ongoing prescription for Dilaudid and robaxin and I hate them! I take the pills only when the pain is so bad that I cannot stand it - this is usually one or two times a month. I prefer me to the pills because I have found Dilaudid doesn't actually relieve my pain symptoms and leaves me nauseous. Robaxin does help, but I prefer mj rather than a pharmaceutical. I would prefer needing none of them and being pain free. I have used mj a couple of times in the past for anxiety and found it to help. Overall, I don't use any one these too often because I have children and prefer to be present, not high. If I use any prescription or mj, I tend to try to hold out until bedtime so that my body/mind might get rest.

1083. Recreationally less problems then alcohol, medicinally less issues with addiction such as benzos and opoid pain pills.

1084. RECREATOINAL MARIJUANA IS A GOOD THING. IT JUST HAS TO BE SEPERATED FROM HARD DRUGS AND LEDALIZED AND TAXED AND SOLD. HARD DRUGS NEED TO BE TACKLED WITH MUCH MORE EFFECT. A 8 YEAR OLD COULD WALK DOWN MY ROAD AND BUY SOME CRACK, WHICH IS REALLY BAD.....

1085. Remember, anything that produces pleasure can become addictive.

1086. Research studies have already shown the great medicinal benefits of cannabis. Alcohol is so much more destructive than cannabis, yet it is legal and in most places cannabis is not. After I drink a lot, the next day I feel horrible, but after cannabis use, the next day I feel refreshed and happy. It's almost as if a cannabis hangover makes my mood so much better.

1087. response depends mostly on energy/fatigue, pain, social context, spiritual/magickal intent.

1088. Rick Simpson oil ingested daily is powerful medicine.

1089. Right now I'm obtaining it through medical avenues but plan to buy recreationally when it becomes available. After not smoking pot for over 20 years and then coming back to it, I've found it to be a very pleasant and helpful experience as an adult who doesn't over-use. I quit two times recently during job searches and it was very easy to quit. The only 'problem' I had was that I missed the pleasant effect of the drug. It definitely helps with social anxiety.

1090. Safer than alcohol

1091. safer than alcohol. some people, not me, are more functional on it. some people think they are more functional, but they arent. and i believe it is a depressant. but it should be legalized.

1092. Same organization that made ir ilegal also wants to make Alovera illegal

1093. Sarcoma patient suffering from PTSD symptoms and anxiety.

1094. sativas and indicas have opposite effects and your choices do not differentiate them.

1095. Seriously considering moving to Colorado because xxx does not even have medical, so as long as I reside here I am truly suffering. I can not afford to continue to fly to Denver to get the MMJ I so desperately need. Porphyria is one of the most rare diseases in the world. There is no cure, and will end my life. With Cannabis I can function, get out of bed, do some house chores and even cook my family dinner. I don't understand why I a,m being forced to suffer in my state.

1096. Short term effects depend on whether indica or sativa dominant is inhaled. I was diagnosed with nervous stomach. No prescription medication has ever worked. I smoke to maintain a certain level of high rather than relieve symptoms as they happen.

1097. Short term effects of marijuana can vary with different strains. Some may make you feel anxious and giddy and other may make you feel relaxed and hungry. Not all effects checked occur with every use. But the feeling of being high is there, sometimes you feel it in your head (sativa) and others in your body (indica). I have been smoking for quite some time, on and off over the years and I would say I do not have any kind of substance abuse problem. I prefer marijuana over alcohol any day due to the physical after effects. There is such a thing as a pot hangover where one may still feel high and a slight headache may be involved. Caffeine (coffee) helps to remedy this. Pot, I belive , helped save my grandmother. She was very ill and frail; significant weight loss and a lack of appetite. Edible brownies allowed her to regain appetite and gain weight allowing for an increase of strength. She has since greatly improved and is living in the community once again. :) happy testing!

1098. Should be avalible in every state.

1099. Should be fully embraced by everyone, has a million uses.

1100. Should be more question about marijuana being an entheogen (spiritual, but not religious).

1101. Should be regulated and taxed. People who consume or grow cannabis for medical or recreational purposes should not be criminals. Weed warriors, while well meaning are ignorant and are participating in a modern day witch hunt

1102. Should be totally legal, and those who disagree are either stupid or evil; and therefore deserving of death.

1103. Should not be illegal.

1104. Sickle Cell Disease

1105. Side effects depend on the strain used.

1106. Simply put;NO HYPERBOLIC RHETORIC: Cannabis&hemp saved my life,which would otherwise be spent in crippling post-surgical pain or addicted to ineffectual opioids and pharmaceutical anti-depressants and sleep aids.I can take care of my wife and home and live a good and functionally 'normal' life as is possible in my circumstances and has far exceeded my expectations of it's effectiveness. I used recreationally in the '70's and basically quit in 1980,using perhaps once every three or more years until 2011 when I nearly died of acute renal failure from overdosing on a combination of my pharmaceuticals and CAT scan contrast. My renal function is normal now and cannabis makes it possible that I can keep them that way. Furthermore,I am fairly well-versed on the endo-cannabinoid system and the role it plays in maintaining homeostasis with the use of supplementary WHOLE PLANT organic phtyo-cannabinoids. Thank you.

1107. Since switching to cannabis I lost 60+ pounds, much happier! no more anti anxiety/depression meds, no more blood pressure meds, migraine meds, pain meds I'm saving money and feel tons better.

1108. Since using cannabis I have been feeling better & eliminated use of RX :) I wish more DR. Would look into this as a better alternative Healthy & no negative side effects

1109. Smoke one and you won't need to be asking... lol No really. I so sleep better and have no trouble taking a leak when I smoke. We all know money is the reason why we can't grow this plant so now the question you should be asking is this... How long will it take to remove the lies about Cannabis from the minds of the people... Have a nice day 3:)

1110. smoke weed everyday

1111. smoke weed everyday

1112. smoked cigs quit 8 yrs ago. Had tumor removed for lung ca in 2012. This very small tumor had been followed for 2 years before surgery was done. Would be interesting to see relationship between heavy mj use and cancer.

1113. Smoked weed recreationally from the time I was 21 to the time I was about 36.n By that time weed got really strong and also expensive. It was easy to just stop using it. Now I am in my sixties, in poor health and a lot of discomfort and pain. I would be happy to just use pain pills like Vicodin, but Drs. won't prescribe it and Cannabis seemed less risky addiction wise, so I researched and decided to take advantage of Medical Cannabis. You need to know that I always EAT my hash oil as the most effective way to deliver pain relief. I refuse to smoke because I dislike the smell, and the mess in my lungs. I use a dab of Cannabis the size of a grain of rice about ever 6 hours and that helps me with pain management without getting me 'high'. If the pain is particularly bad, I increase dosage, despite the risk of getting a strong buzz. A buzz is better than the pain any day. Also, I refuse to drive at all when eating my hash. I see no reason to run any risks of making a driving mistake at my advanced age. Thank you for the chance to share my personal experience of Cannabis.

1114. smoking cannabis greatly improves my ability to focus and visualize my mathematical and scientific questions. I use cannabis before class, tests and homework in order to focus my thoughts on the problem.

1115. Smoking cannabis is a great pain reliever and all around makes me feel happy and content.

1116. Smoking helped in so many ways during both of my pregnancies. With my first one I was sick all the time, smoking helped keep food down. With my second one I had no appetite or desire to get out of bed. Smoking a little bit a day helped me eat and also get out of bed to accomplish my daily tasks.

1117. Smoking makes you surf better

1118. smoking weed has saved my life because it calms me down a lot, especially when i'm feeling suicidal.

1119. so helpful for physical symptoms but really disrupts my motivation

1120. So I woke up last August 2012 with ankles swollen like pumpkins. My eyes were black & blue, & the whites were filled with blood. My bladder was 3 times its normal size, extending up to my belly button and was filled with masses.I had just received an MRI confirming bladder cancer. My kidney's were shutting down and there was no way I was going to go to the ED to let some quack hack on me. Death wasn't the big concern, suffering was. The ER docs would drill tubes into my back/kidneys to drain them & remove my bladder. No thanks. I had previously read about juicing the leaves of the plant for maximum anti-inflammatory results. I was extremely lucky as my friend had just harvested plants. I juiced hundreds of leaves & ended up with 1oz cannabis leaf juice. I drank that @ 9pm. 40 minutes later water started coming out. By 3am, my ankles were skinny again. Impossible! The bladder had to de-inflame to allow water to pass around the masses! I was able to juice for 2.5 weeks, about 1oz/day for 10-12 days. I ran out of medicine. Received emergency surgery 2 weeks later. The masses were highly vascularized & I subsequently bled out, requiring 9 pint transfusion. If I had gotten surgery when I was hyper-inflamed, who knows how bad it could have been. 1 year later, I'm completely pain free for the first time in 15 years. I've been juicing as often as possible, but leaves are in short supply in AZ. Each time I juiced, my joints became progressively less inflamed as I have been suffering from RA-type sxs in major joints since 1st surgery. Oh yea, it solves my cat's leukemia & immunovirus dx. My pts are reporting similar types of profound healing with all preparations (including with their pets). The juice of the leaf is 100, representing awesome. All other intake methods/preparations seem to be 1-5 @ best. That's how powerful the leaf juice extract is! Licensed xx in az. ps: use a wheat grass juicer

1121. So many reasons point to legalization and how beneficial cannabis can be to someone. The fact it's not completely legalized by now is so confusing.

1122. Socially formed and maintained habit! Sustained use for me personally comes from friend group use. Occasionally, I have the infrequent desire to be high alone at home or out and about.

1123. Some answers will depend on type of cannabis you are using and how much you put in a joint or bowl, also there should be a question on dependency rather than addiction

1124. Some folks only use it to accentuate things. If I smoke while things are going well, things generally seem better. If I smoke when I'm depressed (clinically), cannabis tends to make things worse

1125. Some of my friends do show signs o dependence because they need to smoke all day just to get through it. They would definitely be categorized as functional stoners but I on the other hand am not. That's why I rarely smoke and probably why I don't enjoy it very much anymore.

1126. Some of the questions asked are hard to generalize by a yes or no answer. Such as does mmj make you energetic or lazy?

That depends on the strain. I tried to answer the questions on a most of the time basis. If you get a lot of conflicting answers, like checking both the increases motivation and decreases motivation box, then It's because the effect depends on the strain. Also The questions about paranoia and anxiety are hard to answer, If I use mmj and then get paranoid about cops is it the mmj to blame or the laws? In other words people only relate paranoia with using mmj because it is illegal, or not socially accepted. Yes it's still federally illegal.

1127. Some of the questions don't really apply too much - for example, amount smoked per week. Sometimes I don't smoke at all, other weeks I smoke a lot. It depends if I'm stressed, financial situations, and if I'm going to be socialising. For example, if me and a group of friends go out drinking, I would rather smoke a couple of joints at home and only have one or two drinks out.

1128. Some of the questions need a few more options to be more specific

1129. Some of your questions are hard to answer and may show conflicting responses due to the use of different strains in different situations. For example: I use sativa while working, and indica at the end of the day.

1130. some people get confused what the definition of being addicted is. I have friends say that they are not addicted that they just like to smoke, but then they say they cant do certain things without being high. They need it to feel normal is what they say in their words.

1131. Spent all of my life struggling with migraines and insomnia.

Often found migraine medications to be completely ineffective. Insomnia medications were too intrusive on my life. Never pursued any medications for depression or anxiety due to the many unwanted side effects I see them have in other people. Using Cannabis changed my life for the better. My mood is much better, I sleep well, and for once I have a way to handle my migraines consistently and effectively.

1132. Started for anorexia secondary to bleeding ulcers at 18yoa.

1133. Starting to use concentrates more(oils,tincture).

1134. Stress was not on the survey, I use cannabis when I feel too much stress. I take care of my 92 year old mother and it can be stressful. The time of day I usually smoke is in the evening after my mother goes to bed. Another effect I notice is my eyesight is more in focus when I smoke cannabis

1135. Support sensible drug policy.

1136. Survey doesn't provide any type of option referring to physiological vs psychological addiction.

1137. Testing the difference between Cannabis treated with chemicals and Cannabis grown all natural.

1138. Thank you :)

1139. Thank you for creating this survey. In addition to helping me quit alcohol, cannabis helped me quit a 20+ year pack a day cigarette habit.

1140. Thank you for doing this research.

1141. thank you for doing this!

1142. Thank you for taking the time to understand medical cannabis. Like anything else in the world, marijuana use is subjective and is not for everyone. It is 'addictive' only to those who mistreat it and don't respect it for what it is. To a lot of us (and myself), it's a simple natural supplement that hasn't harmed us and only makes life's experiences brighter and better. I really enjoyed this survey.

1143. Thank you for the survey! Peace, happiness and ganja!

1144. Thank you for using 'cannabis' and not the racial slur. We must stop spreading the 'Reefer Madness' lies, and that begins by putting Cannabis & Hemp back into our countries economy. The Hemp market will be great then the medical & social cannabis market combined.

1145. thank you for your efforts to better understand the use of cannabis in WA.

1146. Thanks

1147. Thanks for doing this research.

1148. Thanks for doing this, it's important to de-stigmatize the use of cannabis through increasing understanding. I consider it to be a sacrament, soothing my physical body and enhancing my sense of connection every single day.

1149. Thanks so much for doing this research, it is much needed and as another passionate person about this subject, I am looking forward to doing what I can to spread the truth about such an incredible plant and its long list of benefits.

1150. That it's not harmful

1151. The ability to grow and process cannabis into many forms of food and medicine saved my life. I did not want to be here on this planet, in pain and yet doped up on pharmaceuticals, and almost took my own life because of the pain from being hit by a station wagon at the age of 13, several other accidents at others hands, and several abdominal surgeries. My son is a xx year old, 6 year survivor of xxxxxxxxxxxxx leukemia, and xxxxxxxxxxxxx lymphoma. He also uses cannabis instead of narcotics for the residual symptoms of 6 years of conventional cancer therapy.

1152. The addiction I feel is more psychological & habitual than physical as a change of routine can allow me to go for periods without using it.

1153. The answer choices to the question, 'In selecting my Cannabis medicine I consider these to be important factors:...' is quite limited. Oftentimes, the choice comes down to what is available on the street (I would think this is true for most people). Please consider adding this optional answer

1154. The applications of cannabis greatly vary depending on the strain. Indicas may make you feel much different than a pure Sativa and vice versa, not only in the high but the medical benefits and mood. Many people usually lean towards one or the other depending on personality Indica can be very sedating and calm, almost floating, Sativa on the other hand can be very giggly, euphoric, and uplifting in an inspiring way.

1155. The Best Pain medication for me.

1156. The Cannabis plant has literally saved my life.

1157. The cannabis use pattern section doesn't allow for multiple responses. Very curious to see the results of this survey!

1158. The challenge of stopping cannabis depends on the persons personality/train of thought, weed enhances feelings, if your happy then you will get the giggles but if your sad you will get depressed when under the influence. If you have no issues in your life then weed is easy to stop but when you have issues, weed helps to escape them so that's when it becomes hard to stop

1159. The choices I selected for 'short-term effects immediately after cannabis use' may be contradictory, but I find that the strain of cannabis really makes the difference. Some strains are really uplifting, energetic, and clear-headed versus some are to much of a cerebral high that can make me anxious/paranoid. Other strains are relaxing and euphoric, or couch-lock and stupid. You can be very giggly and super social or 'stoney' and introverted. Not to mention some have dry eye, cotton mouth, or munchies, all of these or none of these. There are so many strains and it seems each person has a different preference. As far as the addiction goes, I generally don't think it is addictive or exhibit any kinds of withdrawal symptoms, however I do think their are people with addictive personalities that can get addictive to weed just like any other abuser (drugs, food, shopping, gambling, etc.). What I can say for sure, is that I can definitely see the benefits when using medicinally for depression, anxiety, nausea, headaches and/or pain. On the other hand, I can also see the benefits for recreational use for positive social appeal, if your an artist, or want to become more focused. All in moderation is key. I hope this helps.

1160. The choices of the effects of cannabis can be both, at times, creative or not, active or not, dependent on idica or sativa. I've put in both of the activities since they apply. It is does not change me all that much. Thank you for doing the survey!

1161. The drug treatment I received was not related to cannabis. Depending on the kind of cannabis I smoke I feel different emotions and have different motivations (ex: exercising vs. listening to music, eating vs. going to a social event, etc.)

1162. The effect on cannabis on me is extremely varied. For instance, if I am feeling anxious before I smoke, smoking will increase my anxiety level. However if I smoke right after a yoga class, smoking helps me have deeply spiritual experiences. If my intention is to right a creative paper, smoking will help me increase my creatively and flow of ideas. So it will always heighten the state or intention I already have.

1163. The effects greatly depend on the strain and method used for intake.

1164. The effects imparted by cannabis run in both directions. If one variety for one person at one time of day on one specific body chemistry profile has a specific effect (ie anti-anxiety), another variety under the same conditions (or changing the other factors) can result in an opposite directed effect (ie increased anxiety). Herbal cannabis more effectively replaces a whole handful of pharmaceutical drugs that each individually have more negative effects than cannabis does. IT IMPROVES HEALTH!

1165. The effects of cannabis vary considerably based on both the strain of cannabis and the users physiology and mindset. I've used cannabis to manage a variety of different ailments over many years with very good results. But the dose and type of cannabis needed has ranged remarkably from high doses of indica (10+g/day) when grappling with chronic pain, high stress life circumstances, suicidal ideation, and devastating IBS flare ups to small, occasional doses of sativa (<0.5g/day) for pain and stress management. So there is no normative patient or dose in the way there is for other medication (cannabis being a modulator rather than a stimulant or depressant). The specificity of strain effects and circumstances that require consistent large doses are reasons why personal cultivation is a critical component of medical access. Most will prefer the variety and guidance available in a dispensary setting, but once you've figured out what works (after a too-long process of suffering through medications that don't), there is substantial benefit in being able to provide it for yourself. Thanks for asking, and good luck with your project!

1166. The experience of being 'high' engages me in the practice of mindfulness. I am able to perceive everything about the present moment and myself in the present moment with 'wider eyes.' This has facilitated deeper appreciation of my life 'as it is now,' and has allowed me to derive deeper value and meaning to the simple (but vital) aspects of my life. In addition, I find that I am always encouraged (after a 'high' experience) to delve deeper into self-care practices. Often, experiencing a high allows me to see mundane truths as profound truths. The necessity for optimal self-care practices and the value of tranquil and peaceful/relaxed interactions with others has become much more concrete to me. I have become better able to understand and more open to cross-cultural viewpoints on health and healing. For me, experiencing and exploring altered states of consciousness is vitally important to my overall well-being. I have found that being able to go into a different realm (or get 'high') has decreased the monotony of everyday tasks. My approach to everything has become infused with a little more life, as I experience profound appreciation (likely due to the mindfulness of a high experience) in the seemingly small, but brilliant areas of my full life.

1167. The first amendment guarantees the freedom to choose how, where, and when one worships.

1168. The frequency of use question is strange to me. I don't always have reliable access to Cannabis, as I don't like interacting with drug dealers and I don't like to burden friends with acquisition. My frequency is more like a couple times every day for a couple of weeks and then nothing for a month or two. Sometimes I use alcohol when I don't have Cannabis. I almost never use the two at the same time. Mostly when I drink alcohol it is because I like it, but right after I run out of Cannabis I might drink a few evenings over the next week.

1169. The gap between medical cannabis and traditional herbal medicine needs desperately to be bridged. Cannabis should be included in healing remedies, alone or in conjunction with the herbs, vitamins and supplements available at any health food store

1170. The introspection I did as a result of cannabis use has been a huge part of saving my marriage.

1171. The loss of short term memory is often wrongly associated as a negative side affect. However when you are trying to relax, the ability to easily drift into another trail of thought is relaxing. Also this survey is flawed and hasn't been thoroughly tested before release. There are several questions where all the options haven't been considered. Like the option to select you don't drive and how some of questions include number ranges too broad.

1172. The majority of recreational smokers who smoke large amounts of weed typically buy through medicinal dispensaries via friends with medical cards

1173. The older I get the less paranoia I experience while smoking Cannabis.

1174. The only addictiveness is mental.

1175. the only thing wrong with marijuana is that it's illrgal

1176. The outcome of short term affects that were listed earlier in the survey depend on the type of strain and if the cannabis is sativa or indica dominant. People may react differently to each type. Some may get super sleepy after using a sativa dominant strain, while others may enjoy it very much. Some people experience paranoia with one type but not the other. When users are first introduced to cannabis and the knowledge of different sativa/ indica strains and how they affect the user isn't known, they may have a bad time and not know why. It's all about finding what works best for the individual's body and mind.

1177. The plant is great to be grown for the help it does to the environment not just ourselves and we need to stop grwoing such a great plant with fertilizers and other 'organics' I just want to juice it but I can only realy get it through smoke so I choose when I do so for I can only grow a tiny plant then juice it and wait till I find a seed in my bag and grow again

1178. The plant is too versatile to be criminalized. Its better to outlaw prescription meds

1179. The quality of my life would be much worse without Cannabis. It has kept me from developing Glaucoma, reduced the amount of insulin I take in my insulin pump on a daily bases. After my 2nd back surgery, and permanent sciatic nerve damage, Cannabis keeps me moving and able to move. It helps with the diabetic neuropathy in my feet and legs. When I am stressed and my blood sugars go on a roller coaster ride, smoking Cannabis calms me back down.

1180. The question about getting in a ticket or in an accident while high is kind of loaded. If you smoke almost every time you leave the house you're bound to be high when you're pulled over, sooner or later, regardless if marijuana had anything to do with it.

1181. The question on short term effects or being stoned was the most difficult to answer I have smoked hundreds of different types of cannabis that have produced all the different effects listed. There are some very bad varieties on the black market that will cause one to feel all the worst symptoms you've listed such as paranoia, anxiety, confusion, dizziness etc. Also being in stressful or non supportive environments while high can also cause these negative effects, having options to buy quality cannabis and to partake in the comfort of one's safe home allows for more positive experiences. I stress that cannabis is addictive because I have tried to stop smoking many times in my life to no avail. I feel completely torn between imagining the positive effects of not smoking, and experiencing the positive effects of smoking. Cannabis has not had severe negative impacts on my life but I somehow feel I could be more productive without it. However the times that I have stopped smoking I have not proven to be considerably more productive, many times it has been quite the opposite. Many of my 'bad' habits which I tend to blame on cannabis use, (such as procrastination, or lack of motivation or productivity) do not improve when I stop smoking. This leads me to think that the problem, if there is one is not caused by Cannabis. Overall I don't consider myself to be lazy or unproductive, it's just that it always seems one could be doing more than one is. On the other hand I don't see myself as an average person. I do and think outside the 'box' if you will, in many ways I think my cannabis use has a lot to do with that aspect of myself. I don't think I will ever stop smoking and I don't think Cannabis has affected my life in any significantly negative way. Thanks for doing this research..

1182. The question(s) regarding cannabis's addictive qualities are too vague. I do not believe that cannabis is physically addictive; the only physical effects brought on by withdrawal of use come from preexisting ailments that were treated with cannabis usage, and psychological effects of ceasing use. However, I believe cannabis to be psychologically addictive, especially to those with addictive tendencies (those more likely to gamble, eat, etc.) I feel psychologically addicted, but I can cease use when I need to (to look for jobs, when I can't afford it, etc). However, cannabis usage does not cause me problems at this time, so I use regularly.

1183. The reason my answers are 'all over' the place is that depending on the strain of cannabis you use, you can experience any and all of those clinical signs. Overall, cannabis has helped me control my pain, and control my anxiety and mania. It has improved my quality of life, and allowed me to stop many harmful behaviors and begin new ones. I am the healthiest I've been in a long time, as well as the most active. That is partially thanks to my cannabis usage.

1184. The reason why I didn't answer the personal driving questions is because I don't own a car. I use marijuana to replace ibuprofen use.

1185. The short term effects are based on whether indica or Sativa is being used and needs to be revised on this survey.

1186. The short term effects seem to depend on the type of cannabis used and how 'stoned' a person is to what really creates their experience I think. I have never experienced any withdrawal symptoms when I go without cannabis.

1187. The short-term effects listed don't always occur - some occur more frequently than others. I just checked off any I have personally experienced as a result of cannabis use.

1188. The Side Effects of the Painkillers, Antidepressants and other prescription drugs I used were really bad. Cannabis had no side effects and worked much better for my PTSD,Anxiety,Depression, attention deficit hyperactivity disorder and agoraphobia. Marijuana gave me back my life quality. Without Cannabis I would not be able to leave my House because of my agoraphobia.

1189. The substance abuse class was court order for a minor in possession of alcohol charge, not related to cannabis. I smoked a bowl before I took this survey.

1190. The survey didn't ask if cannabis helped with creativity or insight, or it's ability to help focus the mind during meditation. It seems the survey covered more myths about cannabis than what really occurs. Like asking if a person feels they are addicted to cannabis. There is no addiction to cannabis. The body requires CBD's to function properly. This is a craving like being hungry or thirsty. We crave what the body needs. Are we then addicted to food and water as well? the question should not have asked if they felt they were addicted but asked if they felt they needed it like being hungry or thirsty. Everyone would have selected that one. So apparently you young people don't truly understand the effects.

1191. The use of Cannabis and it's effects of different people are different. The few that I know that were paranoid or drove poorly after consuming, discontinued use of cannabis because it wasn't fore them. The most I know who do use it, use it for pain, relaxation, and even to motivate when cleaning, reading, or just before exercising. Driving is the most complicated to analyze. I believe it depends on how much has been consumed.

As well as other aspects like if they have had food, water, and enough sleep. I always feel safe to drive, but I only consume small amounts. I know others who can consume large amounts and still drive just fine. The one thing my concern is, in High Schools it's still being sold. I live by a school and I've alerted the school of drug sales right down the street on the corner, in suburbia, and nothing has been done. The younger kids have a higher risk than older people. Thanks!

1192. The use of different strains of marijuana can be used for different health issues, I use cannabis for pain, but also for anxiety and PTSD symptoms. Depending on which issue I'm addressing, my cannabis purchases may differ greatly. This is the same for my domestic partner and many of my friends who are also cannabis users.

1193. the use of medical cannabis has allowed me to regain a significant amount of mobility, allowing me to hike and enjoy the outdoors in the incredible state I live in.

1194. The vast majority of cannabis users are normal members of society and their use does not draw the attention of the law, or others because for most there is no outwardly noticeable effect. As a society we tend to focus on those that abuse substances, whether it be cheeseburgers, alcohol, or cannabis.

1195. The view of cannabis use must be taken in context, n other words, the lifestyle choices of the user must play a significant role in the determination. This is a criticism of mine for too many things these days, Evidence is presnted in isolation but the universe and everything in it is connected not isolated. Nutrition plays a HUGE role in life too as well as the mental state and nutrtion can even play a role on that! Cannabis is medicine that everyone should have access too, we should all be encouraged to grow it! Thanks

1196. The war on drugs needs to end.

1197. There are 3 reasons that restrict my use: employment drug screens, availability, bad product

1198. There are a lot of 'sometimes' answers possible. Should leave more 'other boxes' and you might get more personalized data by putting boxes to 'please explain' answers.

1199. There are a lot of scammers selling oil from hemp seeds as 'CBD oil'. People need education to be able to tell when they're being scammed. People need to look for products that have been tested and use quality controls in manufacturing.

1200. there are more pros to cannabis use than cons

1201. THERE ARE NOT ANY NEGGATIVES OF THIS PLANT!

1202. There are only two options for sex on the survey, you should at the very least provide an 'other' option or maybe just more genders.

1203. There are still millions of people who believe that people who smoke weed will get mental health problems, but I think more needs to be done to prove that while cannabis might amplify an underlying mental illness, it doesn't cause one. We need to basically unprogramme peoples brains to stop believing the decades of propaganda demonising and criminalising a super plant that could single handedly bring down the big pharma companies and solve a lot of problems.

1204. There is a minor discrepancy in your survery. The following question has the Yes and No swapped positions. This may lead to some users to click No, although they meant Yes. The question is: In your opinion, do you believe that Cannabis is addictive? No Yes I don't know All other question have Yes, then No. Just letting you know :)

1205. There is no proof behind cannabis prohibition and no official study or review of literature which demonstrates other than benefit from its use, including during pregnancy, labor and nursing. The entire prohibition is politically manufactured to safeguard private fortunes and consolidate political power.

1206. There is no shame enjoying Cannabis recreationally.

1207. There is so much info on why it should be legal and proving all the superstitions wrong, it speaks for itself.

1208. There needs to be a differential set between recreational and medical users. I consider myself both. I am a 21 year old female, mother, fiancÃ©, living in Seattle. I was diagnosed with ulcerative colitis, major depression, and anxiety. I use Cannabis on a daily basis. I ingest it in a tincture form, which allows me to add it to any food, or just to take it orally. There are no prescription drugs that help me, Cannabis is my medicine. I also use Cannabis to allow myself to 'feel good' from a recreational stand point. I know the difference between the two. I use a tincture that is grown and tested from a collective here in Seattle which is high in CBD. This chemical helps with my pain, like no other. My doctor prescribed me Cannabis that is high in CBD. To use recreationally, I might decide to use a strain of medicine that is a bit higher in THC to give me some euphoria. I believe there are true medicinal values to the Cannabis plant and one chemical that causes euphoria shouldn't disclose that. If recreational users want to get high, they will find a way. Recreational users should just have safe access and just not the same access as medical patients. Because let's face it, a patient with cancer should have more choices of medicine, regardless if it's alternative or not. Recreational users need not all the options on ingestion and limit potency. I think it's pretty Simple, there are medical patients using it as medicine and recreational users, using it to get a buzz. Please help define the difference for everyone else. Cannabis is not just some dried up,crushed up, oregano smelling stuff at the bottom of a plastic baggy, it's a plant. That needs soil, light, and water to grow. It's a plant I ingest for medicine. And it works ! :) thank for reading.

1209. There needs to be a section, and criteria based on college students or your information may be skewed. For instance, I don't really work, which in turn is shown in my small income. Furthermore, I don't drive, nor do I have a licence, something that many people from the city tend to not have, because it is not needed.

1210. These plants are obviously generous gifts to mankind, yet millions face retribution, often violent, for cultivating or possessing cannabis. Many people claim that they have been cured of various serious illnesses with the help of cannabis, yet few jurisdictions will allow them to be prescribed or otherwise legally obtain their vital medicine from this amazing plant.

cannabis can save the world and should be completely legal.

1211. they are distinctly different- the recreational stores do not have the products or quality needed for medicine. Personally, we have developed strain specific glycerine tinctures for pain, sleep, and anxiety. None would be found in a rec store. Also, rec stores allow up to 200 chemicals to be used in growing and we use only organic material...

1212. They are two separate categories that should be allowed to coexist in law.

1213. Think about trying to figure out how to capture the stress and horrors of it being illegal. the worst time for me was having to deal with the lawless issues that are associated.

1214. This drug is everywhere. I strong feel it hold be legal and treated as alcohol.

1215. This herb is one of the most safest and versatile in it's use. Prohibition on the use and cultivation of mmj or hemp is immoral.

1216. this herb revolutionized my life. i'm glad, so glad i see it for what it truly is - Gods gift to mother earth and humankind. peace!

1217. this is cool

1218. This is great. Although in the experience of being high section I realized that there were factors within the experience. For example, at night I would have a different experience then starting off my day with a session. It would be nice to be able to include notes with each question.

1219. This is the most important, useful, and healing plant/medicine of our time. The many uses of all of it's parts can save humanity and the world.

1220. This marks my 49th year of using cannabis. I think it helps me physically and mentally. I am very fit, in part because cannabis helps me exercise. My memory seems sharp, both long and short term. Cannabis also helps me control glaucoma.

1221. this medicine has gotten my sister off of Oxycontin/codone. her quality of life is greatly improved. I use cannabis for pain, but I also use extracts for their preventative properties

1222. this plant has been a godsend, it's has helped me through plantar's fasciitis. i was taking ibuprofen numerous times throughout the day. since i began using cannabis (3 puffs 5 or 6 times a week) i have cut my intake of ibuprofen down to about 2 doses a month. my liver likes that. also, strangely enough, i no longer have a taste for beer, which i use to drink 4-5 a week. i've probably only had 3 or 4 since last year. not sure what the connection is there.

1223. This plant has changed my life! I wouldn't be who I am today had I not come across it's vast range of benefits. I was a slow starter in life. Often sick as a kid too. I grew up in a broken home with parents from widely varying cultures, which was sometimes hard. I developed severe anxiety issues by my mid to late teenage years bordering on agoraphobia. Nature was also kind enough to hand me genetics from both parents who were (cigarette) smokers from an early age which lead to persisting lung problems including severe bronchitis and asthma. I started smoking cannabis in (tobacco infused) joints for the past decade on and off depending on where in the world I happened to be (some places are stricter than others). Since then, my mental and physical health has soared to the point where friends and family have noticed many positive changes. It truly is nature's most healing and versatile gift to humanity. Although, we must be careful as all things have the potential to be abused and overdone. Although overuse of cannabis has hardly any adverse effects (perhaps some paranoia and shivering at worst), too much of a good thing can be detrimental. In my opinion, one should use this plant to the point where it helps them physically and psychologically overcome the challenges of daily life and to improve and enhance their experience on this planet in general - but not to the point where they stay essentially stuck to their couch (or bed) most of the time, doing nothing else but constantly getting high all throughout the day. That would be quite a waste of a life, I think. I hope this helped. I doubt I'd have been able to be so expressive if I wasn't enjoying a mellow, creative Sativa while I took part in this survey. All the best!

1224. This plant has so many benefits physically and emotionally and at least for me I see no side effects unlike all prescription medications.

1225. This plant should be legal everywhere. God provided mankind with this plant for our use. It improves my quality of life tenfold but I live in fear of being prosecuted for using an 'illegal substance' in the state of Oklahoma.

1226. This profile is not capable of accuracy due the issue of availability and affordability. I would have entirely different results if product varieties were reasonably available.....and where it is legally available versus the illegality and criminality of a 'black market'. Political abuse of authority over my decisions of health care choices is not covered within this survey.

1227. This reduced my debilitating medical issues, got rid of my 3 tumors and stopped the seizures and adrenal fatigue symptoms. I feel more functional, excited about life and finally am out of pain so I can create and explore my life! I am so thankful for the difference this plant made for me.

1228. This survey has a typo of sorts. Please see Cannabis Use Pattern

1229. This survey is flawed in its design. It suffers from a voluntary response bias. If you don't know what that is. Hire someone who knows how to design and conduct a proper survey

1230. This survey is very broad on cannabis, cannabis has many uses but having the right flower for its use is important, I know in UK the black market mainly sells strong indicas, a good smoke for night time, but for many people its all they get, so they smoke it in the day also. Therefore my answrs may seem somewhat contradicting at times, this is the reason for that. The next point is in UK its very likely to get contaminated cannabis from the blackmarket where you get addicted to something you dnt even know you are smoking. Ive experienced bad withdrawals with these, but good cannabis is usually fairly easy to take breaks from. Another point I dont see covered nearly anywhere is that in countries where it is illegal to consume, people live in a life of fear, fear of meeting a criminal once thats over then fear of getting caught by police on your way home, then to be in fear of your parents finding out. In these years i was more anxious and paranoid. Once I had a good source that was dropped to me and my parents were aware of my habit those problems are moreless non existent

1231. This was so intertwined with our culture since the dawn of civilization. It was highly likely to be the very first crop sowed by man. It was greed and hatred that made it illegal. We need it back. Our bodies want it back. Our body has receptors specifically for cannabis. Receptors that help regulate our health. Give us cannabis back.

1232. This whole topic is so complex; it's difficult to to find the right words; especially because this plant means so much to me. I think that Cannabis has so many different medicinal values. It could replace (most) painkillers, antidepressants, sleeping pills, antiepileptics, appetite stimulants, chemotherapy and so many more. The highest medicinal values for me personally are definitely the psychic ones. I can say that it saved my life more than just once. But I would also like to treat my grandmother's cancer with cannabis oil after I watched my other grandma die from it and the chemotherapy. The most improtant thing about the use of cannabis is education. I really don't like the fact that so many (young) people misuse this wonderful plant. Another problem are the (illegal) commercial growers. They only have one goal: Highest THC levels for maximum psychedelic effects. That's not what it's supposed for. After I had to stop growing my own Cannabis I had no other possibility than buying from a dealer. I had to quit quite soon because I experienced extreme paranoia (caused by high THC and low CBD levels and especially the law (mostly the thought of being caught, getting arrested and losing my driving license caused those negative effects)). I'm very sad about it because it helped me a lot. To conclude: We definitely need a legalisation for medicinal purposes and controlled growing. Recreational use by the age of 18 would be ok, too. Cannabis is definately not suitable for minors (but they should rather use Cannabis than alcohol, tobacco etc.) I'm interested in the findings of this survey, so if it is possible I would be pleased if you can send them to me via email. I'm also interested in participating in further surveys concerning Cannabis. Thank you for your work on this topic.

1233. Though cannabis may cause 'anxiety' , I think it is due to the accurate perceptions of other dimensional interactions, or the spirit world that is being seen or heard.

1234. time permitting, i can smoke from once a month to once a day

1235. To elaborate on the whether or not marijuana is addictive, I would like to say that the plant itself is not physically addictive, rather emotionally addictive to some individuals. It is an incredibly versatile plant whose legality can and hopefully will benefit us all. It is refreshing to see legitimate research being done so as to avoid the stigma around this subject!

1236. To keep the studies about this great natural medicine,

1237. To so many of the questions in this survey. It depends on the strain of the Cannabis you use. And depends on the mood the person is in for the type of 'high' they are looking for. Good luck with your findings, peace x

1238. Topical salve has cleared acne

1239. Topical use is wonderful for joint pain and discomforts.

1240. Treatment for substance abuse was a series of classes after I got 2 DUIs almost ten years ago. Since then, I never ever drink alcohol and then drive. I will often use cannabis while driving. It hinders my ability to drive only in that packing the pipe diverts my attention from the road.

1241. Under amount used I left it blank because I only use cannabis concentrates. I smoke about 4-7 grams of hash oil per week.

1242. Unemployed but I am a university student.

1243. Use Cannabis for degenerative disc disease.

1244. Use cannabis to help me gain perspective of what i want and feel because when i smoke i can more easily separate what others think and want me to do and what is true to me.

1245. Use of cannabis varies from user, environment, social situation (or non-social). When addiction is mentioned above it would be nice to differentiate physical and mental addiction, considering the physical addiction of marijuana is rare on light users or even non-existent. Especially comparing them to tobacco or alcohol. Also, when asked about tobacco use, consider asking and understanding how many people smoke marijuana mostly in tobacco blended ways - 'spliff' or half marijuana, half tobacco water pipe 'hits.' It'd be very interesting to one day see the effects of marijuana smokers that ONLY used cannabis and no tobacco products.

1246. Use this data and publish it please, we all are curious and hopeful, mostly curious. Thanks

1247. used cannabis while in extreme pain with pregnancy - no evidence of negative affect on baby - unless her charming happiness was a result...

1248. used primarily as a social activity at first, later used for stress release/sleep/libido and for the enjoyment of the altered mental status associated with use (increased awareness of connectivity/patterns, humour!)

1249. Used to just smoke now I work with patients and the oil.

1250. Using cannabis has allowed me to function better day to day, less pain, less muscle spasm, less anxiety. It also allows me to control my medications more fully.

1251. Using cannabis improves my quality of life to no end. My biggest issue is how stigmatized its use is - even in my family still. Let's get this work done to help patients and destigmatize this flower

1252. Using Cannabis makes my life more bearable, I have spent decades taking pharmaceutical drugs to no avail, I am deemed 'drug resistant'. The pharmaceutical drugs (especially anti psychotics) cause awful side effects such as massive weight gain and heart problems!) cannabis causes me no side effects and my physical health has improved by 80% since giving up pharmaceutical drugs and using cannabis instead. My mental health has also improved because of this. Unfortunately, in the UK the government hides it's head in the sand and is insistent that cannabis has no medicinal relevance whatsoever,the media demonises it and the police and courts sentence people for being found with as little as a gram or growing one plant, this is despite the well known fact that millions of people use it in the UK and many grow their own for medicinal purposes..

1253. Using it nightly after dinner/before bed helps me 'shift gears' - I calm down, relax, am less 'snippy' with my teenager (who may/may not know I use MMJ - I've never 'come out' to him - fwiw: he's staunchly anti-drugs of any kind - largely because he hates his ADHD meds and believes people should be 'natural' <shrug>), and I sleep much much better. On weekends, I'll sometimes use a saliva blend to better motivate me to do household chores and yard work. Again, it makes me feel more chill/mellow, and able to focus on the tasks at hand.

1254. Using methods such as vaporizing and edibles greatly diminish if not eliminate the negative effects of cannabis on the human body long term.

1255. Varieties high in thc and low in cbd tend to cause anxiety. When any variety is harvested late (over mature) it has a sedative effect. Edibles that are heated too hot or too long are extremely sedative and can be psychedelic. 180 degrees f for one hour seems to be best for edibles.

1256. Very concerned about the impact of new recreational laws on medical. To the point of tears. Haven't purchased medically but know many who do and the taxation will be unaffordable to the point many will go without medicine they need.

1257. Very context-dependent drug. If stressed in work/life, then will be anxiogenic. If relaxed or happy in life, can be a very enjoyable experience. Irritability results if have to be responsible within 24-48 hours, so rare use (limited to Fridays and sometimes Saturdays). Smoked regularly before becoming a professional and parent (with attendant stress of school, finances, responsibilities).

1258. We are at the infancy stages. MMJ will help you reach further and learn more about you on the inside.

1259. We are made for cannabis(endocannabinoid system). It can be made for medicine,food,fuel,material,clothing etc. It needs to be legal in all states so we can cure ALL diseases.

1260. We need more honest and informative education concerning both the benefits and drawbacks of cannabis use. Cannabis really isn't a problem. Starvation, war & inequality are problems. Get it legalized/taxed and move on to bigger issues.

1261. We should be bound as a family on earth to understand what harms us and keeps us together working optimimly.

1262. We should regulate. Cannabis is a medicine and a gift from nature

1263. We should treat medical and recreational use of cannabis separatly (in regard of the law). I use cannabis mostly for medical use but enjoy the side effects. I also appreciate the passion some people have behind the plant, from growing a great quality product to extracting the purest medicine. It is some sort of applied science. :)

1264. We stopped allopathic meds 5 years ago. We are very happy utilizing natural remedies.

1265. we want cannabis to be viewed as a medicine not a recreational drug.

1266. Weed is awesome man

1267. weed is great

1268. Weed is just misunderstood! legalize it!

1269. Weed is legal where I live. I enjoy that weed is legal where I live. I also smoke weed that people have grown themselves.

1270. Weed isn't addictive it's how weed makes you feel that you are addicted to!

1271. Well for one they need to hav part Indian to chk I'm German / American Indian I smoke weed both for th high n th medical benefits I don't like Man made pills they all hav awful Side affects alot r poison I am ADHD hurt my back severely yrs ago it's so bad can't b a union carpenter anymore that's y I Wrk part-time now th only thing that gets me threw th day is my weed it's a life savior

1272. Well I've smoked since 76 the days if 400 a # COLUMBIAN GOLD nd hash oil I use because I love it an feel so much better after use. Alsoused caused of CMT charcot marie tooth.

1273. Well the question about short term side effects, there are so many different answers since it all depends on the strain. Different kinds do different things.

1274. What a beautiful herb! Grateful the world is finally realizing its benefits and harmlessness, even it's ability to reduce crime and rates of alcohol use. Thanks for studying this!

1275. What completely skews research and what you should definitely, definitely take into account is how different cannabis can be. A chunk of indoor, hydroponically grown, stinking, indica, 20% THC 1% CBD bud will have a completely, COMPLETELY, different effect to a chunk of light, outdoor grown, sativa hash (5% THC, 7% CBD). I cannot express quite how different it is. The effect of cannabis on the mind is also hugely, hugely dependent on the mind in question, pre-cannabis. It effects everyone very, very differently, and someone's 'personal effect' can vary hugely. Sometimes cannabis makes me motivated, creative, outgoing, happy, and relaxed. Sometimes cannabis makes me socially awkward, quiet, introvert, and a little anxious (this is why I have sometimes ticked contradicting boxes). Unfortunately the latter is more common than it has ever been, although still uncommon. I think I may have just smoked a little too much weed, basically, it's lost part of its fun. That's why I'm reducing my intake, which I'm having no problem with. A problem I have is that I, pardon my French, fucking LOVE smoking my pipe. The taste, the action, the culture, I adore it. So I find that often my urge to smoke cannabis is for this pleasure, and not to get stoned. And it isn't some psychological addiction kicking in telling me that, I know when I want to be stoned - I often turn down people's 'twos.' It really is just because I enjoy smoking the pipe. I now smoke herbal cigarettes (Greengo) to try and combat this urge to smoke, which does help. I think the simple act of inhaling smoke is a little addictive in its self. Also on the topic of addiction, please please please take into account tobacco use - for three years I was one of the millions that smoke their herb with tobacco, but never cigarettes. As a regular user I obviously got addicted to the nicotine, meaning I had to smoke spliffs regularly or get nicotine withdrawal symptoms. In the process of quitting tobacco I learnt an awful lot about nicotine and the subconscious - I really think a lot of so called cannabis addiction is really just tobacco addiction. But even those that plain cigarettes too, surely taking a very addictive drug (nicotine) EVERY single time they use cannabis, without fail, will skew the brain's idea of cannabis? Especially if they really enjoy the effects of cannabis? Anyway, you've read this far, congratulations, and I'm sorry for writing all this - I hope it wasn't too soul-crushingly boring. Good luck with your research etc. If you feel you'd benefit from contacting me, I have an awful lot to say on the subject - I'm in a bit of a rush and I'm not satisfied with what I've written here (I'm better than this, I swear!). My email address is xxxxxxxxxxxxxxxxx Please feel free to pass on my email address to any law enforcement agencies it may concern. Seriously though, happy researching. See you on the flip side.

1276. When asking if cannabis is addictive, you should differentiate between a chemical dependency and psychological addiction. I know from personal experience you cannot be dependent on it but do believe you can be 'psychologically addicted'

1277. When I am dealing with major intellectual problems I will use cannibis to help me see the bigger picture or force me to look at it from angles I may have been subconsciencely ignoring. I was addicted to marijuana for 4 years while living in Colorado during prohibition and absolutely had difficult getting away from it. This also considering I was a 24/7 user. Doing anything 24/7 would likely be difficult to stop. Now that I am older I get more paranoid after use as I now worry about being able to handle my responsibilities while impaired

1278. When I am using cannabis it helps with my chronic lower back pain and other issues I experience throughout the day. If I am doped up on prescription drugs things are not as clear and I still hurt alot.

1279. When I began upgrading my cannabis consumption from recreational to medicinal, my chronic cervical spine pain began to get better,, which is awesome because the doctors were trying to push me into surgery. I no longer take any prescription pain meds. I only take IBU200's when I absolutely need them (once a week if that). On the addiction side of it, I don't think anyone ever quits a 'habit' without the irritable effects of 'changing.' It sucks, but if you have ever seen REAL WITHDRAWALS from people with REAL ADDICTIONS, hearing the word addicting and cannabis in the same sentence is a slap in the face. EVERYONE IS ADDICTED TO CANNABINOIDS, and obviously, the longer you go without something your body needs, well, you are going to suffer. I went to jail for 90 days for a Driving on a Suspended. Within the first week, the pain was back. The cold concrete cell and steel bed probably didn't help matters, but the pain became unbearable by week 2. I would eat a couple of Tylenols and actually feel a buzz as the pain lifted away from my neck. Painlessness is bliss. But then it came back, usually with a little more veracity. So quitting 'Marijuana' is a bullshit lie that assumes the user would be better off if they didn't use the substance - ALL THE WAY TO PUTTING YOU IN JAIL TO PROTECT YOU FROM A PLANT? What you really make people do it to discontinue a vital supplement that is actually preventing people from getting ailments,

1280. When I first started smoking Cannabis I sometimes had negative symptoms like intense anxiety (which was a pre-existing issue for me) or difficulty with short-term memory, but now that I've been using Cannabis for many years it combats my issues with anxiety and I now encounter almost no negative symptoms (other than the occasional dry mouth) in my daily use.

1281. When I go on a period of not using canabis, I normally get very vivid dreams for the next few days. I also believe that whether or not it impairs your ability to drive should not interfere with whether or not it gets legalized federally.

1282. When I have an IBS flair up the only thing that will help is cannabis. Sadly in New Zealand we can pick and choose what cannabis we buy and it's always usually indica which is terrible when you want to get stuff done. So it's a win lose situation for me. I also suffer from depression and anxiety and sometimes cannabis can make it better and sometimes worse as I can get a bit paranoid and room bound but that maybe because of the strain... but I'm unsure as we're not sure what were buying.

1283. When I said it was not addictive, I meant that it wasn't, under the right circumstances. Moderation in all things is key.

1284. When I say it addictive I don't think it's addictive like cigarettes (I smoke years ago, I quit 9 years). But I miss it, physically and mentally.

1285. When I tried pot in college it was a joint and I did not feel a thing; i realized much later that it was because I had never smoked anything (cigarettes or otherwise) and didn't really know how to 'inhale.' Edibles make it much easier to control how much I use when I do use it, which is still recreational and still relatively infrequent as compared to others I know. I am forwarding this survey to everyone I know that currently uses though since I know several that are regular users, for both recreational and medicinal purposes. I really appreciate that research is finally being done.

1286. When I use cannabis it calms me down, helps me focus and it gives me that cloud nine feeling that couples get when they're in love.

1287. When I was 12 yrs old, my family doctor prescribed a nerve med because I wasn't handling my parents divorce well. I took that med for over a year and hated the way it made me feel. I then started using marijuana and quit the prescribed med. the marijuana helped me so much without the 'icky' feelings (both mental and physical) that the prescribed meds did. I have been a steady user since and frankly am tired of having to 'hide in the closet'

1288. When I'm sad I smoke, when I'm happy I smoke, when I want to go out and have fun I smoke, when I want to stay in and have fun I smoke. I smoke when I don't feel well. I'll even smoke when I'm frustrated with something then I can usually sift through my feelings and make logical statements about my frustrations that help me even in the long run.

1289. When severely depressed, cannabis can keep people from doing stupid things.

1290. When smoking only at night, ie. 1-3 bong hits before bed, I find that the cognitive effects of Cannabis are relatively few.

However, when I smoke Cannabis starting in the afternoon, with one bong hit, I find myself to be less thoughtful. Also, my intent with Cannabis use is to reduce my thoughts and slow my brain down. It does this fantastically. I find that Sativa strains do not have this effect, rather these strains make me extremely thoughtful. I think you should also know I am a full-time student with a double major, two research assistant positions, and an internship that requires 15-20 hours a week from me. I'd say I function excellently for my status. In addition, both of my parents and several adult family members consume Cannabis on a daily basis. Each of these individuals are considered to be top performers in their respective industries (government defense contracting and/or environmental engineering).

1291. When you guys ask about 'addiction', you should do it less ambiguously. For instance, I smoke in a daily basis because it makes my life so much better than it was before. I'm happy now. I could leave it easily, without crisis like other physically addicting drugs, I just chose not to :) on the other hand, I'm pretty sure none of my aunts could ever leave coffee for a day.

1292. Whether it's indicated and saliva alters dramatically my highs- one makes me energetic one makes me lazy as fuck

1293. While I believe marijuana is not inherently addictive, I do believe that the human mind can become addicted to anything. As such, recovery systems should be in place for those looking to seek them out. I have used marijuana as a spiritual aid to help with the introspection needed in this age, an age where no one has time to sit with themselves. I continue to use it to this degree and fully advocate its use as a medical aid to understand the underlying psychological causes of depression and anxiety.

1294. While I don't believe that marijuana is physically addictive I do believe that it can be psychologically addictive to I some people. I believe that marijuana can be an extremely effective treatment for PTSD in particular. I had tried many medications before marijuana to ease my symptoms, but there is no pharmaceutical drug that has ever been able to relieve my symptoms as quickly and thoroughly as marijuana.

1295. While I feel I've become 'dependent' on cannabis, I don't feel that it's addictive. I can go a whole day with out cannabis and be completely fine, days even, but I'll still want to smoke when I can!

1296. while I have heard repeatedly that pot isn't addictive my husband acts like an addict and his use keeps increasing. He complains of severe muscle twitching when he tries to stop. I don't really know if it is withdrawal or a problem because of the nerves irritated in his back.

1297. While I have not used Cannabis for my melanoma (I'm in remission), I have the MMJ authorization so that, should a new lesion develop, I can quickly go on Rick Simpson Oil. My research suggests that 'ethical pharmaceutical' alternatives are both ridiculously expensive and, effectively, ineffective. My oncologist, upon questioning, admitted that cutting it out of my body was the only effective treatment for this cancer.

1298. While I think that cannabis can be mentally addictive, I do not think it can be physically addictive. Also would be interested in potential effects of cannabis on a baby during pregnancy to alleviate symptoms.

1299. While I was consistently using Cannabis I had received the best grades I had ever gotten in a semester of college, with more rigorous coursework. I had the ability to better focus and organize my thoughts. I was able to write papers efficiently and effectively where I used to struggle before. I felt that my papers sounded more intelligent when I wrote them high. Additionally, I felt that I had become more open-minded to thoughts and ideas, really beginning to find myself. I became more of a critical thinker, and I was able to concentrate on one topic for a long period of time exploring endless possibilities. Cannabis has made me feel connected, more loving, and peaceful. Pure bliss. I found my spirituality while using cannabis, and now believe in and practice exercises I never thought I would.. such as yoga, and meditation. Overall I feel happier and healthier than I've ever been. I have experienced anxiety while using cannabis occasionally, not every time. I believe that's because I was using more than one to three times a day, every day. So I simply cut down my use without any 'withdrawal' symptoms. At first I was a little more irritable, but that was short lived and it is so easy to stop using whenever I desire. I don't have to have it I just enjoy the positive benefits, which significantly outweighed the negative, every so often. I am still very motivated, and in the best shape I've ever been in. I will be successful in life, and I don't think cannabis has negatively effected me in that aspect in any way. I also want to point out that Cannabis has been proven not to have a significant impact on lung function, but rather slightly elevates lung function. Thank you.

1300. While not chemically addictive, I strongly believe the lifestyle of chronic recreational cannabis users can have negative effects. This includes decreased motivation to function in society and poor physical conditioning. However, a vast amount of

Americans would be able to benefit greatly from the occasional use of cannabis.

1301. With long term use I find it to be addictive and have mild withdrawal symptoms. It is important to learn and control your tolerance especially if used for medical reasons. It however does wonders for my Irritable Bowel Syndrome and appetite issues and if I find the right strain it really can help anxiety.

1302. With sufficient cannabis of the appropriate strains - I will be returning to work after 20 years of disability ... as xxxxxxxxxxxxxxxxx of a Licensed Commercial Provider (Lic under Health Canada) producing and dispensing meds to patients with either ATPs (Authority to Possess - 'license' under MMAR) or Rx (under MMPR). xxxxxxxxxxxxxxx is poised with the most advanced (Copyright and Trademarked) systems proprietary strains plus huge funding reserves to be Canada's #1 provider of medical cannabis and reserch and development.

1303. with the general exception of adolescence- the only thing that compels a person to get 'high' on cannabis is free will- Also, it is an unnatural state for our species to NOT have a medical/industrial/recreational relationship with cannabis- cannabis is likely the most beneficial vegetable known to science

1304. With use of cannabis, I am able to hold down a full-time job, something that I can't do on the medications I would need to control my medical issues. Without cannabis, I'm in too much pain to support my family. Without cannabis, I spend my days in bed, sick and in constant pain.

1305. without the use of cannabis I would be dead ,in prison and on americas most wanted list !

1306. xxxxxxxxxxxxxxxxxxxxx. Good luck with your research.

1307. Yes I admit that cannabis can be addictive, but it is a VERY small chance of addiction forming.

1308. You asked if I believed pot to be addictive. I answered no because I don't believe it to be addictive physically but I have experienced psychological addiction.

1309. you didn't differentiate the method of cannabis consumption in regards to driving time. for example i would never drive within 2 hours of eating an infused edible, but i would drive within 2 hours of smoking. you didn't quantify if any other stimulus was contributing to mental health issues or if mental state was typical for the subject or not. that would probably be helpful since i personally tend to use cannabis more to help cope with stress and less when i am not under much stress.

1310. You guys are doing a great thing, keep up the excellent work. –xxxxxx

1311. You have a lot to learn in a respectful meaning! Most of the people on the boards regulating this industry, and most all medical professionals are clueless on this subject. Wish I could help conduct your data quest, you need experienced professionals to get the correct info.

1312. You have a research design flaw: the initial questions do not specify whether you want quality of life, etc, with or without cannabis use. My answers describe life since I have been using cannabis medically, but my answers would be enormously different if I was telling you what life was like *without* medical cannabis.

1313. You might reconsider your categorizations of gender to be more inclusive. Participation in a 12 step recovery program is not a proxy for addiction as many 12 step groups address situations with food, sex, co-dependency, etc. Finally, there was not an option to convey that I do not drive at all, regardless of my cannabis use. Thanks!

1314. You need to have multiracial as an option if you are going to use a single select on the ethnicity question.

1315. you need to know the quality of the cannbis i smoke is what i class as top quality, well cured and flushed plants with a good genetic strain and knowing the difference between body and head highs

1316. You should ask these questions of people who are not currently smoking/using cannabis, or who rarely use it.

1317. You should know that if people like and want to smoke a plant, we will. regardless weather the government thinks they can control that or not! Its my body and I choose what goes in it! Good or bad!

1318. You should know that it being illegal is hurting and putting people in a worse place than to what the would be if it was legal is natural it's on the planet for a reason why should we not be aloud consume it weather it's medical or recreational

1319. You should know that you are doing an awesome thing here. I love seeing more people doing research on one of the earths greatest herbs. Please keep in mind that a 'hit' off a vape can vary significantly depending on the vaporizer. You may ask how much cannabis is used and how toasted the cannabis looks after the session. There is also the question of how much edible cannabis a surveyor is consuming. Edibles also vary a lot in the potency or dosage.

1320. You should look into how people smoke more.

1321. You should make the ethnicity boxes multiple choice... Or include a 'mixed race' option. It's 2014.

1322. You're only a lazy stoner if you're a lazy person. I'm extremely kind, generous, intelligent, successful, funny, and happy. Cannabis helps me a lot, and if it affected everyone negatively, I wouldn't be able to say those things truthfully. I'm glad to see the public is finally tired of being lied to.

1323. Your questions about how you feel after smoking are misleading - it depends on the strain. Many patients, like me, will have their day-time strain, evening-time strain, special pain management strain, or even an anytime wellness strain. With one strain, I may feel energetic and motivated and less of an appetitie, and another I may feel couch lock and sleepy and have the munchies, and then sometimes I have a high CBD, low THC just for wellness that doesnt seem to effect me at all right after.

1324. Your survey asks 'How long do you typically wait before driving following Cannabis use?' I chose one hour after cannabis use. The survey then asked 'Do you believe Cannabis impairs your ability to drive safely?' I chose sometimes. It is important to note that I rarely feel impaired by cannabis and if I do feel impaired I don't drive. Cannabis does not affect my ability to determine if I can safely drive. I can reason out whether or not I am too impaired to drive.

About the Authors

Michelle Sexton received her ND from Bastyr University and completed a postdoctoral fellowship at the University of Washington in the Departments of Pharmacology and Psychiatry and Behavioral Sciences. She is the Medical Research Director at the Center for the Study of Cannabis and Social Policy. Her NIH-funded pre-doctoral and postdoctoral research was on the topic of the pharmacology of cannabinoids and the role of the endocannabinoid system in neuroinflammation and neurodegeneration. Her postdoctoral project was investigating the potential role of cannabis use on endocannabinoids and inflammatory markers in patients with Multiple Sclerosis.

Dr. Sexton serves as an editor and technical advisor for the American Herbal Pharmacopoeia Cannabis Monograph. Dr. Sexton has presented her research internationally and is published in peer-reviewed journals. Dr. Sexton's clinical practice, research and teaching focus includes treating clinical endocannabinoid deficiency and the medical use of cannabis across a range of conditions and age groups. She is a member of the International Cannabinoid Research Society, the International Association of Cannabinoid Medicine and the Society of Cannabis Clinicians. She maintains a small medical practice in San Diego, CA.

Laurie K Mischley, ND PhD MPH studied naturopathic medicine (ND) at Bastyr University and epidemiology (MPH) and nutritional sciences (PhD) at the University of Washington. Her work is focused on identifying the nutritional requirements unique to individuals with neurodegenerative diseases. She has published on coenzyme Q10, lithium, and glutathione deficiency in Parkinson's Disease (PD).

As a clinical researcher, she has worked with the FDA, NIH, and the Michael J. Fox Foundation to administer intranasal glutathione, (in)GSH, to individuals with PD. Drawing on expertise in radiology, epidemiology, nutrition, neurology, and naturopathic medicine, she is attempting to determine whether (in)GSH boosts brain glutathione and improves health.

She has served on the Bastyr University Institutional Review Board since 2010 and regularly provides integrative medicine research mentorship to students. She founded the Social Purpose Corporation, NeurRx, developed an outcome measure to assess PD severity, www.PROPD.org, and is author of the book, *Natural Therapies for Parkinson's Disease.*

Dr. Mischley maintains a small clinical practice at Seattle Integrative Medicine focused on nutrition and neurological health.

Acknowledgments

Many thanks to
Bastyr University,
The Cannabis and Social Policy Center (CASP),
Coffeetown Press,
and all the people who responded to the survey
for making this book possible.

INDEX

EDITOR'S NOTE: Because the flavor of the original responses has been preserved by not correcting misspellings, some responses may not be included in the index.

www.ingramcontent.com/pod-product-compliance
Lightning Source LLC
Chambersburg PA
CBHW011829020426
42334CB00027B/2985

* 9 7 8 1 6 0 3 8 1 6 1 5 1 *